ETHICAL FOUNDATIONS OF HEALTH CARE

Responsibilities in Decision Making

Jane Singleton, DPhil, BA
Senior Lecturer in Philosophy
University of Hertfordshire, UK

Susan McLaren, PhD, BSc, RGN
Senior Lecturer, Department of Nursing and Midwifery
Director of Undergraduate Nursing Studies
University of Surrey, UK

Mosby

London Baltimore Bogotá Boston Buenos Aires Caracas Carlsbad, CA Chicago Madrid Mexico City
Milan Naples, FL New York Philadelphia St. Louis Sydney Tokyo Toronto Wiesbaden

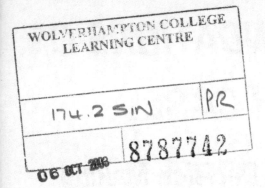
Publisher:	Griselda Campbell
Project Manager:	Louise Crowe/Jane Hurd-Cosgrave
Production:	Joe Lynch
Index:	John Gibson
Cover Design:	Lara Last

Copyright © 1995 Times Mirror International Publishers Limited

Published in 1995 by Mosby, an imprint of Times Mirror International Publishers Limited

Printed in England by J W Arrowsmith Ltd.

ISBN 0 7234 1873 X

For full details of all Times Mirror International Publishers Limited titles, please write to Times Mirror International Publishers Limited, Lynton House, 7–12 Tavistock Square, London WC1H 9LB, England.

A CIP catalogue record for this book is available from the British Library.

Contents

Preface

The Importance of Ethics

Ethical questions are central to health care practice. What is a just allocation of health resources? Who ought to receive treatments if resources are limited? Ought we to use eggs from aborted fetuses for infertility treatments? Ought requests for voluntary euthanasia be granted? Under what circumstances is it justifiable to use individuals for medical research? Who ought to take health care decisions? These examples, which are by no means exhaustive, are illustrative of the important dilemmas that are faced in health care.

It is important to realise just how pervasive ethical issues are. Even the naming of the recipients of health care as 'patients' or 'clients' has ethical implications. Accordingly, throughout this book the authors have used the term 'individual' to refer to the recipient of health care in order to avoid prejudging the nature of the relationship between health care practitioners and the recipients of health care.

The Purpose of the Book

In addition to being designed as a foundation textbook for all health care courses and applied moral philosophy courses, a feature of this book is the authors' argument for the positive thesis that decision making in health care should be a matter of participation between members of the health care team and the individual receiving treatment. The importance of the autonomy of the individual is taken as central and a paternalistic model of decision making is rejected. This centrality of the consumer in the decision-making process highlights the importance of a consideration of the rights of individuals receiving treatments.

The Structure of the Book

It is argued that a knowledge of ethical codes of conduct is not sufficient to answer the sort of important ethical questions illustrated above. Rather, a detailed analysis of the **Principles of Autonomy, Justice, Beneficence** and **Non-maleficence** are needed to assist reflection on these issues.

These principles and the differing justifications that are offered for them within consequentialist and deontological theories are considered in Section 1. Section 2 of the book considers the detailed application of these principles to contemporary health care dilemmas. The first part of this section addresses life-and-death issues and the second part concentrates on issues of daily practice. Within these sections, Jane Singleton, a lecturer in philosophy, wrote Chapters 1–11 and Susan McLaren, a nurse, wrote Chapters 12–17. This combination of two disciplines is seen as particularly valuable in this area where both an understanding of the philosophical issues and an awareness of health care practice are crucial.

In order to assist cross referencing between the philosophical discussion of the ethical principles and their application, a numbered system of cross referencing is used. The first number refers to the chapter number and subsequent numbers to the sections within that chapter. In addition, certain material is repeated in order to clarify the exposition.

Where philosophical theories are considered in Section 1, quotations from primary sources are used to allow the reader to evaluate these positions in their original form. This also removes the necessity for consultation with extra texts.

Several other features are included to assist in the use of this book as a textbook. Learning outcomes and exercises are placed at the beginning and end of each chapter, respectively. Important definitions, summaries of points and questions have been emphasised by including them as key points at the end of each chapter. In addition, at the end of the book, there is a glossary of philosophical and health care terms and appendices which include The Patient's Charter, various professional codes of practice, research guidelines and UKCC advisory papers on important ethical questions.

Case studies are used to provide illustrations of the points that are being made, but they are not designed as highly detailed examples. More information would be needed for decisions to be made in the majority of these examples.

SECTION I

PHILOSOPHICAL FRAMEWORKS

Introduction

'The important thing ... is not so much to obtain new facts as to discover new ways of thinking about them.' [1]

Learning outcomes

After reading this chapter, you should be able to:
- Recognise when ethical issues arise in cases.
- Provide a critical analysis of ethical codes.
- Understand the meanings of the *Principle of Autonomy, Principle of Beneficence, Principle of Non-maleficence* and *Principle of Justice.*
- Be able to recognise when appeal is being made to these principles.
- Have an initial understanding of the relation between ethics and the law.

1.1 ETHICAL ISSUES

Most people would claim that they can recognise an ethical issue. They realise that ethical questions, such as 'ought one always to tell the truth' or 'are abortions ever morally justifiable', are different from factual questions such as 'how much is your tax bill' or 'which is the quickest way from London to Edinburgh'. However, it will become apparent that we need to look more closely at these ethical questions in order that we can think more clearly about the issues involved and the ethical decisions that have to be taken in health care practice. What is an ethical issue? What distinguishes ethical questions from other sorts of questions? Here are three examples within which we can identify some ethical issues.

The mother-to-be example

A 39-year-old female undergoes an amniocentesis. The results indicate that the fetus is not suffering from certain genetic abnormalities. The mother requests to know the sex of the fetus. This information is refused on the grounds that an abortion might be requested if the fetus is not of the 'right' sex.

In this example, questions requiring expert medical knowledge would have been raised when considering the advisability of offering this test to the patient. Medical expertise is also required to be able to interpret the results of the test. However, ethical questions also arise at both these stages. Should the life of the fetus be put at risk by undertaking this test? If the test indicates genetic abnormalities, is it justifiable to abort the fetus? Is it legitimate to withhold information gained from this test?

The euthanasia example
A 70-year-old widow in agony from rheumatoid arthritis decided she wanted to die. The request was judged to be competent and was agreed with by her only son. The doctor gave her an injection of potassium chloride and the widow died some minutes later. A member of the nursing staff wonders whether to report the consultant's action.

In this example, medical knowledge would be required to diagnose the woman's condition and realise its prognosis. Additionally, it raises ethical questions. Is voluntary euthanasia morally acceptable? Since it is illegal, should the consultant have agreed to the request for euthanasia? Would it be right for a member of the nursing staff to report this action?

The pain-killer example
A consultant has decided that a patient has become too dependent on certain pain-killing drugs that will ultimately have harmful consequences. It is decided to wean the individual off these drugs without informing her. The nurse is required to continue this deception even though the patient is clearly distressed and asks why her pain killers are not having their usual effect.

In this example, we have a judgement based on medical knowledge that the pain killer will ultimately have harmful consequences. We also have the assessment that a weaker pain killer will be adequate to deal with the particular complaint. However, the ethical question arises of whether or not one should deceive this individual. In addition, the nurse in the health care team might not agree with this deception, so should the nurse tell the patient the truth or should she continue the deception ?

1.2 ETHICAL EXPERTS?

One of the things that these examples illustrate is that the expertise required for diagnosing, treating illnesses and caring for individuals is not the same as the expertise needed for taking ethical decisions. A skilful health practitioner is not necessarily one that is equally skilled when ethical decisions arise. It must not be assumed that, because we consult someone about a medical complaint, that person is also the one who should take ethical decisions when they arise. Our argument is that solutions to ethical problems in health care are not the prerogative of health care professionals. Rather, solutions to ethical problems rely on participation between the individual and the health care team. We shall be analysing these ethical issues to assist both health care workers and other members of the community in their consideration of ethical questions.

'1.3 PATIENTS' OR 'CLIENTS'?

When discussing the sort of ethical questions illustrated in our examples, we must be careful not to beg any important ethical question in our description of the cases. In the 'pain-killer example', the individual has been referred to as a patient. The term 'patient' has the value implication that the relationship between this individual and other members of the health care team is one of dependence. This relationship of dependence, implied by the use of this term, might go some way towards justifying the paternalistic course of action taken in this example. We need to be able to consider the ethical questions raised by this case using terms that do not automatically favour one course of action over another.

Instead of the term 'patient', it might be thought preferable to use the term 'client'. This does not appear to have connotations of dependency and gives the recipient of health care more autonomy. However, if the term 'client' is used, then this carries implications from the business field into the health care relationship which again begs important ethical questions. For example, is it appropriate that the availability of certain treatments should be based on the ability to pay just as business services are open to those who can afford them?

Therefore, we need to find a term to refer to recipients of health care which is not too cumbersome and which does not beg the question in favour of certain ethical conclusions. Accordingly, in this book we refer to the recipients of health care as 'individuals', which appears to be the most neutral term from a value point of view. In calling them individuals, no value issues governing their relationship with members of the health care team are presupposed.

1.4 ETHICAL CODES

If we return to the examples with which we started, it might be argued that we already have a way of dealing with the ethical questions that they raise. We can refer to the ethical codes of practice that apply to the different members of the health care team and argue that these provide guidance about what ought to be done in cases like these. For example, there is the ethical code produced by the United Kingdom Central Council for Nursing, Midwifery and Health Visiting. This provides a list of clauses for the conduct of nurses, midwives and health visitors in their relationship with the recipients of health care, other members of the health care team and any other relevant bodies. As an illustration, one of these states that they should:

> 'Act always in such a manner as to promote and safeguard the interests and well-being of patients and clients.' (See Appendices for ethical codes governing practice.)

However, there are a number of reasons why referring to ethical codes of this sort will not provide solutions to the type of ethical questions illustrated in our examples.

Meanings of key terms

The first difficulty is to understand the key terms used in the list of clauses. In the example given above, what counts as the 'well-being' of an individual and who is to determine whether the individual is in this state? What is meant by the distinction between 'promoting' and 'safeguarding' well-being and interests? Until these terms and others like them have been explained, the meaning of the code will not be clear (see 15.3.4).

Conflicting requirements

A second problem with the codes of practice is that the requirements within them do on occasion conflict. For example, another clause from the code just quoted states that carers should:

> *'Work in a collaborative and co-operative manner with health care professionals and others involved in providing care, and recognise and respect their particular contributions within the health care team.'* (See Appendices for ethical codes governing practice.)

In the 'pain-killer example' the nurse might well feel that there is a conflict between the requirement in the first clause that we quoted to promote the well-being of the individual and the clause to work in a collaborative and co-operative manner with other members of the health care team. Consulting the first clause alone might lead the nurse to think that it is right to tell the individual about the deception that is being practised. However, the second clause would appear to advocate continued concealment on the grounds that this is what constitutes co-operative behaviour with other members of the health care team.

Not exhaustive

A third problem with relying on ethical codes for the solution of ethical questions is that ethical codes are not exhaustive. They do not provide clauses to cover all the ethical dilemmas that might arise in health care. Many examples illustrate this point, but 'the mother-to-be example' illustratesit particularly well. It is clear from the code to which we have been referring (see Appendices for ethical codes governing practice), that there are no clauses that indicate what ought to be done in this case. Who, for example, is to be considered the patient/client in this case? Was it in the interest of the fetus that the amniocentesis was undertaken or in the interest of the mother? Whose interest is being considered when the request for information about the sex of the fetus is refused? Even when these questions are answered, the clauses by themselves do not provide an answer to our ethical questions.

No justification

Another problem with the expectation that ethical codes might provide solutions to ethical questions is that they are just presented as lists of clauses. They provide rules for the ethical conduct of a nurse, midwife or health visitor but there is no indication of what the rationale for these rules might be. What principles are being employed to arrive at these rules? Are they principles with which the nurse, midwife or health visitor would agree? Although these codes clearly provide some level of guidance, without an appreciation of their rationale they cannot be used as a substitute for making ethical decisions.

This problem is not limited to codes for nurses, midwives and health visitors. It also applies to the Hippocratic Oath and the various codes issued by the World Medical Association. Similarly, other health care practitioners, such as physiotherapists, have rules of professional conduct which are subject to the same criticisms (Rules of Conduct for Physiotherapists are issued by the Chartered Society of Physiotherapy).

Acceptability of the codes

A final problem is concerned with the acceptability of the codes. Up until now, we have been writing as though the codes might provide some guidance in ethical decision making but are by no means sufficient in themselves when dealing with complex ethical questions. However, it might be worth remembering that these codes were not devised by consulting many different sections of the community but were devised by a minority group from within the community. For example, the United Kingdom Central Council for Nursing Midwifery and Health Visiting has a committee that is responsible for the production of the code for professional conduct. Although every nurse has a right to vote for members of this council from which the committee membership is formed, this does not guarantee that the resulting codes and free from flaws. There is no reason why communities should accept uncritically codes that have been established by a minority group. Indeed, the requirements incorporated in the Hippocratic Oath (see Appendix), for example, might come to be seen as too paternalistic and individualistic. In fact, Veatch writes:

> *'The Hippocratic Oath is dead. No rational person would agree to it.'* [2]

1.5 CRITICAL ETHICAL APPROACH

If ethical codes do not, by themselves, provide answers to the ethical questions, we need to adopt an alternative procedure. A critical ethical approach needs to be taken. This begins by analysing four basic philosophical principles which underlie ethical decision making. In addition, specific issues are analysed where these principles are seen in operation.

Analysis of basic principles

If we return to the examples with which we started the chapter, we might be able to abstract some common principles that are being appealed to implicitly. One such principle is the Principle of Autonomy, that is, the principle that in certain areas an individual has a right to be self-governing. This is particularly evident in the 'euthanasia example' and the 'pain-killer example'.

In the 'euthanasia example', the Principle of Autonomy is being respected since the woman's wish to die has been granted. Presumably, it is also felt by both the consultant and the woman's son that her well-being or benefit lies in this course of action. Thus, the action is also what is required by the Principle of Beneficence, that is, the principle that the well-being or benefit of the individual ought to be promoted.

By way of contrast, in the 'pain-killer example' the Principle of Autonomy is overridden by the Principle of Beneficence. The action is assumed to be for the benefit or well-being of the individual being treated and it is this that justifies overriding the individual's autonomy.

In the 'mother-to-be example', the Principle of Non-maleficence is relevant. 'One ought to do no harm' is a principle that is at the heart of health care. In this case, the possibility of harming the fetus is overridden in favour of what are taken to be the benefits of having the test, or the Principle of Beneficence. A Principle of Justice might also be involved in this sort of case since limited resources might raise the question of who is thought to be eligible to have this diagnostic test. A Principle of

7

Justice that states that equals ought to be considered equally requires analysis in order that we can apply it when the question of distribution of resources arises.

In order to clarify our thinking about the ethical questions we have illustrated, we need to look at these four principles in turn to find out precisely what they mean. This involves looking at how these principles can themselves be justified (see Chapter 2).

Ethical analysis of specific questions

In addition to analysing these four principles, a critical ethical approach will subject specific issues to analysis. In the 'mother-to-be example', the question could have arisen of whether abortion is justified in cases where the fetus is found to be suffering from genetic abnormalities. In analysing this sort of question we shall need to consider questions such as 'What sort of beings have a right to life?', 'What does it mean to have a right to life?', 'Do fetuses have the same rights as other human beings?' and 'When does life begin?'

The 'euthanasia example' raises different issues. We shall have to look at questions such as 'Is any form of euthanasia justifiable?', 'If euthanasia is justifiable, is there any moral difference between killing an individual and omitting to treat?' and 'What is to count as death?'. It also raises an issue of professional practice about what to do when a colleague has performed an action of this sort.

Unlike the so called 'big dilemmas' concerning life and death, the 'pain-killer example' raises questions that arise in daily practice. Questions that would need to be considered are, for example, 'Is there any justification for withholding the truth from individuals?' and 'What principles ought we to use when there is a conflict between duties owed to other members of the health care team and the individual being treated?'

The law

A critical ethical approach to these issues is not restricted to what is, in fact, legally allowed at the present time. We are considering what ought to be the case and this might not be coincident with what is at present allowed by particular laws. For example, in the case of voluntary euthanasia, where an individual requests the termination of his or her life, we shall consider what principles could provide a justification for this and what principles are being employed by those who deny it is justifiable. The fact that voluntary euthanasia is illegal in the UK at the time of the publication of this book does not in itself provide an answer to the ethical question of whether or not it ought to be allowed.

Conversely, if a critical ethical analysis leads us to the conclusion that something is morally wrong, that does not mean that it ought to be legally prohibited. It might be considered that there are certain areas of an individual's life that ought not to be within the domain of the law. Mill wrote:

> 'That the only purpose for which power can be rightfully exercised over any
> member of a civilised community, against his will, is to prevent harm to others.'[3]

If we take the case of voluntary euthanasia again, it could be argued that the individual wishing to die is not harming others. If this is correct, laws would not be justified in this sort of case. Even if voluntary euthanasia were shown to be morally wrong, that would not mean that it ought to be legally prohibited.

Outcome of a critical ethical approach

What will be achieved by a critical ethical approach to these issues? It would be ideal to think that as a result of this approach we could programme the equivalent of an ethics computer and await the solutions to ethical problems. This is not what will be achieved. Rather, the aim is that ethical problems should be clarified by analysing the issues. Analysis will reveal the sort of principles that are implicitly or explicitly referred to in our preliminary look at the examples at the beginning of this chapter. Discussion of principles such as the Principle of Autonomy and the Principle of Beneficence will not provide easy solutions to ethical questions but will assist reflection on these issues.

Arguably, a further advantage of this approach is that greater understanding of these ethical questions will enable individuals to sympathise more readily with ethical positions with which they disagree. For example, when there is a clash between their personal morality and what is required in their professional practice, a deeper understanding of the principles that could underpin positions other than their own might ease the conflict. An obvious example of this is in the area of abortion where personal commitment and professional conduct might conflict.

A secular approach

Finally, although religious perspectives on these issues are considered, the book is concerned primarily with secular ethical theories. This is not intended to devalue a religious approach but rather to reflect the fact that many individuals are now considering these problems outside of a religious framework. In addition, many of these problems cease to be problems if a religious ethic is adopted. Certain problems are solved automatically by virtue of religious principles.

LEARNING EXERCISES

1. Analyse one of the ethical codes given in the appendices highlighting any problems that it might contain.
2. A 59-year-old male needs a heart operation but he is told that he cannot have by-pass surgery until he gives up smoking. The doctor is prepared to give him the operation if it is done privately but he will not perform the operation under NHS funding. The individual cannot afford to have the operation done privately. He agrees to give up smoking but nine months later when he has arrived at the top of the waiting list and is just about to have the operation, the surgeon asks if has given up smoking. When the individual admits that he is still smoking, the surgeon refuses to operate and tells him to rejoin the NHS waiting list. What ethical issues arise in this case and to what principles is appeal being made?

REFERENCES

1. Bragg, W.L. From *Quotations For Our Time*. Ed. L. Peter (1982), Methuen, London.
2. Veatch, R.M. (1981) *A Theory of Medical Ethics*. Basic Books, New York, p144.
3. Mill, J.S. (1985) 'On Liberty'. In G. Himmelfarb (ed.), *On Liberty*, Penguin Books, London, p68.

Key points
- The Principle of Autonomy. In certain areas an individual has a right to be self-governing.
- The Principle of Beneficence. The well-being or benefit of the individual ought to be promoted.
- The Principle of Non-maleficence. One ought to do no harm.
- The Principle of Justice. Equals ought to be considered equally.

CHAPTER 2

Consequentialist and deontological theories

'Both horns of a dilemma are usually attached to the same bull'.[1]

Learning outcomes

After reading this chapter, you should be able to:
- Explain the doctrine of Consequentialism.
- Understand the main characteristics of Hedonistic Consequentialism.
- Understand the main characteristics of Interest Consequentialism.
- Have an understanding of Kant's deontological theory of ethics.
- Describe and evaluate differences between deontological and consequentialist ethics.

2.1 JUSTIFICATION OF ETHICAL PRINCIPLES

In the examples that we considered in Chapter 1, we saw that there are four main principles appealed to in ethical decision making: Principle of Beneficence, Principle of Autonomy, Principle of Non-maleficence and Principle of Justice. In the following example, three of these principles are considered.

The cancer example

An individual has cancer and asks a member of the health-care team, in this case a nurse, what is wrong with him. The nurse knows from close relatives of the cancer sufferer that he will be overcome by depression if he knows the true diagnosis. He has the prospect of a few more months of life with some pain that could be alleviated by drugs. It seems reasonable to suppose that the quality of life of the sufferer in these last few months will be better if he does not know the truth of his diagnosis. Should the nurse tell him what is wrong with him?

The Principle of Autonomy is clearly relevant here. The right to be told one's true medical condition would appear to be an area over which an individual has a right to be self-governing. This knowledge might affect how the individual would like to conduct the last few months of his life. For example, there might be certain things that he would choose to say to those who have been close to him. Also, he might choose to spend the last few months at home, if this was possible, rather than in hospital.

However, it might be argued that application of the Principles of Beneficence and Non-maleficence favour not telling this individual the true diagnosis. It might be assumed that harm would be done to the individual if he knows, since then he will be overcome by depression. Since the Principle of Non-maleficence states that one ought not to do harm, application of this principle would appear to favour non-disclosure. Put positively, the Principle of Beneficence is applicable since the duty to benefit here might be assumed to be accomplished by not telling the individual the truth. Therefore, in this case it would appear that application of the Principle of Autonomy favours a different action to that which would result from applying the Principles of Beneficence and Non-maleficence. Although we have a clearer understanding of the nature of our dilemma by making explicit the principles that are only present implicitly in the description of the case, we have not been able to determine which course of action the nurse should take.

What we need is a further understanding of how these principles can in turn be justified. We need to know what considerations fundamentally underpin the way that we look at ethical dilemmas. For instance, in this example we might say that what we are fundamentally trying to achieve is the best outcome in this case. We want to reach a decision that will yield the best results or consequences for the individual concerned, his relatives and others such as health-care workers involved with his case. This is the essence of consequentialist ethical theories (see 12.3.1 and 12.3.2).

2.2 CONSEQUENTIALIST ETHICAL THEORIES

The view that what is important is that the best consequences are achieved has been formulated by Parfit as:

> '... there is one ultimate moral aim: that outcomes be as good as possible'.[2]

Therefore, in the 'cancer example', we should be asking: 'What will produce the best outcome in this situation?' This is the fundamental question that we need to ask when we look at ethical dilemmas.

2.2.1 Act consequentialism

There are different ways in which we might seek to answer the question of what will produce the best outcome in ethical dilemmas. In the 'cancer example' we might ask directly: 'What is the right action for the nurse to perform?' and not make any reference to the three principles mentioned above. If we did this, we should only consider the consequences on the individual, relatives and other members of the health-care team of the nurse's action of telling or not. The consequentialist view of what would make her action right would be that *an action is right if it produces the best possible outcome.*

If we approached the question in this way, we would first of all have to determine what is the best outcome and then from this it would follow what is the right action to perform. The right action would be that one which would, on this occasion, produce the best consequences. What is to count as the right action therefore becomes something that is dependent on the ethical decision about what is the best outcome. Thus, rightness is defined in terms of what produces good outcomes.

2.2.2. Rule consequentialism

In order to avoid what might turn out to be a lengthy examination in each separate case of what is going to yield the best outcomes, it might be suggested that certain principles or rules could be justified on consequentialist grounds. If this could be done, then when a principle with a consequentialist justification is applicable in a certain case, we would know that adoption of this principle is likely to lead to good outcomes. Instead of applying the consequentialist justification directly to acts, we should be using it to justify certain rules or principles. Thus we have *a rule is right if it produces the best outcome possible.*

In Chapters 4,5 and 6 we shall consider how the Principles of Autonomy, Beneficence, Non-maleficence and Justice might be justified on consequentialist grounds.

Other rules might also be considered as justifiable on consequentialist grounds. Thus, in the 'cancer example', it might be the case that the rule, 'One ought to tell the truth,' has a consequentialist justification. Acting in accordance with this rule is likely to produce the best consequences. If this is the case, the right action to perform from this point of view would be for the nurse to tell the truth. The right action is the one that is in conformity with the rule which has a consequentialist justification.

This way of applying the consequentialist doctrine is indirect, as opposed to the direct application considered in the act consequentialist approach. We are not considering the consequences of an individual action but evaluating an action as right because it falls under a rule that has a consequentialist justification. In the 'cancer example', we are not considering directly the consequences of the nurses action in this particular case. Rather, we are evaluating the nurse's action of telling the truth as being right because the rule, 'One ought to tell the truth', has a consequentialist justification.

What are good outcomes?

Whichever of these two approaches is adopted, the doctrine that outcomes be as good as possible does not give us a complete ethical theory. We need to know what are to count as good outcomes in order to apply either our act or rule consequentialist doctrine. We need to attach a value theory to our consequentialist claim which will tell us what are good consequences.

There are many different views about what are to count as good consequences. These views all claim that what is good is fundamental. That is, no further justification can be given for what is taken to be a good outcome; it just is good. Another way of making the same point is to say that what is good has intrinsic worth. It is not good because of something else that it might yield, it is good in itself.

These views are still described as consequentialist theories but differ in the view they take about what has ultimate value. In looking at these different value theories that can be combined with consequentialism, we do not discuss whether the particular author is applying consequentialism to individual actions or to rules. Our concern will simply be to examine the value theory that is being proposed. Application of these theories to the four principles is considered later.

2.2.3 Hedonistic consequentialism (utilitarianism)

The classic consequentialist doctrine is that put forward by Bentham[4] and later by Mill[5]. Although they put forward different accounts, they agree on the fundamental point that what has ultimate value is happiness. Good outcomes are those that yield happiness. This view has a certain initial plausibility that makes it worth examining. If we take the 'cancer example', we are trying to achieve as much happiness as possible for the individual and others affected in the situation.

Mill wrote:

> 'The creed which accepts as the foundation of morals, Utility, or the Greatest Happiness Principle, holds that actions are right in proportion as they tend to produce happiness, wrong as they tend to produce the reverse of happiness. By happiness is intended pleasure, and the absence of pain; by unhappiness, pain, and the privation of pleasure.'[5]

This is clearly a consequentialist theory since what is right is being determined by the consequences of an action and the consequences that are taken to be good are those that produce happiness. In this initial formulation at least, happiness is being equated with the sensation of pleasure and the absence of pain.

Because consequentialism is here being combined with a theory that states that good outcomes are those that produce happiness, it is called hedonistic consequentialism. Indeed, this phrase is often what is meant by the term utilitarianism and that is how I shall use this term. Mill describes his theory as utilitarianism. He clearly intends to capture by this term that it is both a consequentialist doctrine and one that gives intrinsic value to happiness. However, sometimes the term utilitarianism is used synonymously with consequentialism. This should not cause any undue problems since the context of the use usually clarifies which sense is intended.

One of the obvious features in favour of this sort of approach to ethical problems is that it reduces all issues of value to one common currency of pleasure and the absence of pain .This should, in principle, make it easier to arrive at a solution to ethical problems. The right action to perform will just be that action which produces the greatest balance of pleasure over pain. However, this seeming simplicity masks many problems. How exactly are we to measure these sensations of pleasure and pain? Mill himself argues later in the essay that there are different sorts of pleasure. He describes these as intellectual and sensual and claims that the intellectual pleasures are more valuable than the sensual ones. How are pleasure and pain to be recognised in those individuals who cannot express their experiences?

Mill recognised some of the difficulties with his initial formulation of the doctrine where he equates happiness with the sensation of pleasure and the absence of pain . Indeed, towards the end of the essay he starts to describe happiness as 'a concrete whole'[6] which comprises the concrete things that individuals desire. The individual is happy then in proportion to the amount of his or her desires are satisfied, in proportion as he or she has what he or she prefers. It should be noted, however, that this sort of position is in direct opposition to earlier parts of Mill's essay where he specifically distinguishes happiness from satisfaction or contentment[7].

However, this move away from taking happiness to refer to some mental state of pleasure and the absence of pain to considering it as a reflection of desire satisfaction is what is reflected in contemporary consequentialist theories. These theories, then, are also consequentialist adhering to the claim that outcomes be as good as possible. However, they combine this with a different view about what constitutes a good outcome.

Interest or preference consequentialism

Recent formulations of consequentialist theories take the interest or preference satisfaction of those affected to be what counts as a good outcome. Singer advocates the former view in his book *Practical Ethics* [8] and the latter position is argued for by Hare in his book *Moral Thinking* [9]. Interests are taken to encompass anything that individuals desire. Singer, for example, lists the following interests:

> '... the interest in avoiding pain, in developing one's abilities, in satisfying basic needs for food and shelter, in enjoying warm personal relationships, in being free to pursue one's projects without interference.' [10]

One of the obvious questions with this sort of account is what sort of beings can be said to have interests and are there some interests, for example, in the continuation of one's own existence, that some beings cannot possess? If we consider the beginning of life, can the fetus at all stages of its development be said to possess interests? Even if it can possess some interests, do these include an interest in the prolongation of its life? If the interests of the fetus conflict with the interests of other individuals, how are these conflicting interests to be weighed in order that the maximum satisfaction of interests be achieved?

These difficulties will be raised later when the adoption of interest or preference consequentialism is considered in particular cases. Interest or preference consequentialism is arguably preferable to hedonistic consequentialism, since there are many problems associated with the measurement of the sensation of pleasure which are apparent in the hedonic calculus proposed by Bentham[11].

2.3 DEONTOLOGICAL ETHICAL THEORIES

If we return to the 'cancer example', we might say that what is important to consider here is not what will cause the best outcome. Rather, certain features of the situation make certain actions right or wrong in themselves. For example, one such characteristic in this example might be telling the truth. Although this might sometimes be overridden, the rightness of telling the truth is something intrinsic to truth telling itself and is not dependent on truth telling resulting in good consequences. This is to take a deontological approach, which can be contrasted to the way that the rule consequentialist viewed truth telling (rule consequentialism, above) where the rightness of truth telling was justified in terms of it being instrumental to achieving the best outcome.

Perhaps the major point of difference between deontological ethical theories and consequentialist ethical theories is that the former take rightness to be primary. As we have seen, for consequentialists, what is right does not have any independent standing but is defined in terms of what produces good outcomes. It is then this latter notion that receives an independent explanation. In the case of deontological ethical theories, certain actions are intrinsically right and their rightness is not dependent on some further claim such that they are productive of the best outcomes. In fact, the best outcome will be achieved, in deontological terms, if the right action is performed. This is because the right action determines what is the best outcome. Clearly, if a view like this is held, then some account is necessary of what makes certain characteristics right. Why should something like telling the truth be regarded as something that is intrinsically right? The following deontological theories provide answers to this question.

2.3.1 Kant's deontological ethical system

Just as Bentham and Mill provide the classic statement of a hedonistic consequentialist view, so Kant's ethical theory contains the classic statement of a deontological theory. Kant proposed a test called the 'Categorical Imperative' which could be used to test whether a certain rule, such as one ought to tell the truth, was really a duty (see page 16). The Categorical Imperative is first formulated by Kant as:

'*Act only on the maxim through which you can at the same time will that it should become a universal law.*'[12]

What does this mean? To begin with, what is a maxim? An example of a maxim that we might adopt is that we shall always do the shopping on a Friday. Another one might be that we will always take anything that we want even if it does not belong to us. From these examples, we can see that a maxim is a subjective principle of action. It is a principle that we have decided to adopt to govern our lives. In order to see if our maxims are duties, we shall then have to see if they pass the test incorporated in the Categorical Imperative.

So what exactly is involved in this test? As a minimum requirement for a maxim to be capable of becoming a universal law, a law applicable to everyone, it must not contain contradictions when stated in its universal form. Kant gives an example of a maxim which, if universalised, would be self-contradictory. Let us suppose that we decided to have as one of our subjective principles of action the maxim of making promises which we had no intention of keeping. This could be a very useful maxim for us. For example, I could borrow some money from you and promise to pay it back even though I had no intention of doing this. However, Kant argues that such a maxim could not become a universal law since it would be self-contradictory. He writes:

'*How would things stand if my maxim became a universal law?' I then see straight away that this maxim can never rank as a universal law of nature and be self-consistent, but must necessarily contradict itself.*'[13]

The contradiction present if this maxim is universalised is that the practice of promise keeping would disappear. This is because no one could rationally believe anyone's promises since they would be aware that the other person had no intention of keeping them. To make a promise implies having the intention of keeping it and hence it is contradictory to both have and not have this intention. Indeed, it is difficult to see how there could be these insincere or lying promises unless there were a practice of promise keeping. This is because they derive what success they achieve from the existence of the institution of promising. That is, from the fact that most people make promises with the intention of keeping them.

Although lying promises fail this test incorporated in the Categorical Imperative there are some maxims that are not contradictory when universalised but are still not duties. This is because they fail the second part of the test incorporated in the Categorical Imperative. If we have as one of our subjective rules of action that we shall just look after our own interests and not help others who might be in need of our assistance, could this become a universal law? Kant writes:

> '... it is impossible to will that such a principle should hold everywhere as a law of nature. For a will which decided in this way would be in conflict with itself, since many a situation might arise in which the man needed love and sympathy from others'.[14]

The suggestion here appears to be first that there is no formal contradiction in everyone adopting the policy of just looking after their own interests and not helping others in distress. However, we shall find that we cannot both have this as one of our maxims and at the same time want it as a universal law. That is, we would not choose this maxim and also hold that everyone else should just look after their own interests. The merits of Kant's argument about this point are hotly debated but it is clear that Kant is suggesting a two-part test in his Categorical Imperative since even if a maxim, when universalised, is not contradictory, it does not automatically follow that it can become a law. It has also to pass the second part of the test and be such that we can will it both as a subjective principle and as a universal law.

The necessity of being able to universalise our maxims, of acting as if you were legislating for everyone, is not the only feature incorporated in Kant's account. In formulating principles of action that pass this test we need to recognise that other human beings are also ends in themselves and must not be treated as a means to a further end. If we make a promise with no intention of keeping it then we are using someone as a means towards an end which we desire but which they do not share. Finally, other rational beings as well as ourselves will formulate principles and recognition of this will impose restrictions on what maxims can pass the test of the Categorical Imperative. These last two points are discussed in further detail in 4.2.2 when we consider Kant's justification of the Principle of Autonomy.

If we return to the 'cancer example', the maxim of telling the truth would appear to pass the test incorporated in the Categorical Imperative. When this maxim is universalised and applied to everyone, there is nothing self-contradictory in everyone telling the truth. In addition, if we want to tell the truth ourselves we shall want other people also to tell us the truth. This maxim therefore passes both tests and is thus a right-making characteristic (see 12.3.2).

One of the major problems with Kant's deontological system is that there might well be situations where more than one thing is our duty. This in itself is not problematic except where these duties conflict in the sense that it is not possible to perform an action which is in conformity with both. Arguably, this situation might be said to arise in the 'cancer example' where it might be claimed that the two duties of telling the truth and not harming someone are in conflict.

2.3.2 Ross' deontological ethical system

An account that could remedy this problem was put forward by Ross in two books published in the 1930s called *The Right and the Good*[15] and *The Foundations of Ethics*[16]. Ross proposed that certain duties such as fidelity, beneficence and justice be regarded as what he called prima facie duties. These duties are those that we just, from our ordinary moral convictions, regarded as duties. He recognised that in some situations these could conflict and the duty that was finally decided to be applicable in the particular situation would be regarded as our absolute duty in that situation.

If we return to the 'cancer example' again, Ross might have argued that there are two prima facie principles involved, the principle of non-maleficence, that is, the non-infliction of harm, and the principle of telling the truth. Our ordinary moral intuition reveals that these are prima facie duties and where they conflict, we must somehow find the greatest balance of right over wrong in order to discover what is our absolute duty in this case.

2.4 EVALUATION OF CONSEQUENTIALIST AND DEONTOLOGICAL THEORIES

During the course of this book, we shall see in detail the implications of adopting one or other of these approaches, but I will make a few points now about these competing theories.

Consequentialist theories have what seems, on the face of it, to be an advantage since there is only one thing that is claimed to have intrinsic value. For Mill this was happiness and for other philosophers it was preference or interest satisfaction. Everything of value can be reduced to the one common currency of happiness or interest satisfaction. Consequently, everything of value can be directly compared since all value issues are explicable in terms of one currency. This would appear to make moral dilemmas more easy to solve and less intractable. In the 'cancer example' we would just have to consider the interests of the individuals affected in this situation and the right action to perform will be that action which maximises interest satisfaction.

However, one might have an initial feeling that not all values are indeed commensurable and that any account that claims they are is not reflecting the sophistication of moral thought. Also, despite its apparent simplicity, any account which evaluates actions or rules in terms of consequences is going to have to weigh probabilities of certain consequences against the amount of good that those consequences might yield . Therefore, any calculation might be very difficult to undertake.

Perhaps the most fundamental criticism that can be levelled at consequentialist theories is that separate individuals are no longer of paramount importance in their account. The maximisation of happiness or interest satisfaction is the goal to be achieved. If this is achieved by an unequal distribution of happiness between individuals, then nothing can be done about this. We shall see how this ultimately leads them to give an unsatisfactory account of the Principle of Justice in Chapter 6.

An initial advantage of deontological theories is that they appear to advocate as right what is generally recognised by the majority of people as being right. However, what characterises a moral dilemma is that this is usually a situation in which these prima facie duties conflict. It might be felt that deontological theories do not provide a decision procedure to deal with these sorts of cases. Any talk of 'weighing' the various prima facie duties against one another is not descriptive of a method at all. However, maybe this is all that can be hoped for and after the situation has been suitably clarified, we shall in some sense see what course of action will be right.

The fundamental advantage that deontological theories have over consequentialist theories is their recognition of the importance of individuals. It is not legitimate to sacrifice individuals for the sake of a particular favourable outcome. Our argument is for the importance of this claim throughout the book.

LEARNING EXERCISES

1. 'There is nothing wrong with undertaking a pregnancy with the sole purpose of providing fetal tissue'. What justification, if any, could be given for this claim from within a consequentialist ethic?
2. If three people's lives can be saved by using the organs from a fourth person, ought we to kill the fourth person to obtain his or her organs? Analyse this question from both a deontological and consequentialist perspective.

REFERENCES

1. Kohn, R.M.H. (1970) *Perspectives in Biology and Medicine*, Sumner Press, p633.
2. Parfit, D. (1984) *Reasons and Persons*. Clarendon Press, Oxford, p24.
3. Bentham, J. 'An Introduction to the Principles of Morals and Legislation'. In M. Warnock (ed.) (1968) *Utilitarianism*. Fontana Library, Glasgow.
4. Mill, J.S. 'Utilitarianism'. In M. Warnock (ed.) (1968) *Utilitarianism*. Fontana Library, Glasgow.
5. *Ibid*, p257.
6. *Ibid*, p 291.
7. *Ibid*, p260.
8. Singer, P. (1933) *Practical Ethics*, (2nd edn). Cambridge University Press, Cambridge.
9. Hare, R.M. (1981) *Moral Thinking: Its levels, Method and Point*. Oxford University Press, Oxford.
10. Singer, *op.cit.*, p31.
11. Bentham, *op. cit.*, pp64–5.
12. Kant, I. 'Groundwork of the Metaphysic of Morals'. In H.J. Paton (ed.) (1948) *The Moral Law*. Hutchinson University Library, London, p84.
13. Kant, *op.cit.*, p85.
14. Kant, *op.cit.*, p86.
15. Ross, W.D. (1930) *The Right and the Good*. Oxford University Press, Oxford.
16. Ross, W.D. (1939) *The Foundations of Ethics*. Oxford University Press, Oxford.

Key points

- Consequentialism. There is one ultimate moral aim that outcomes be as good as possible.
- Act consequentialism. An action is right if it produces the best outcome possible.
- Rule consequentialism. A rule is right if it produces the best outcome possible. This can be determined by considering the question, what would happen if everyone did this sort of thing. For example, possibly a rule such as 'One ought to be honest' could be justified on the grounds that if practised generally this would yield a good outcome.
- Hedonistic consequentialism. Outcomes are right in proportion as they produce happiness and wrong as they tend to produce the reverse of happiness. Happiness is understood as the mental state of pleasure and the abscence of pain.
- Interest consequentialism. Outcomes are right in proportion as they produce the satisfaction of the interests of those affected.
- Categorical Imperative. 'Act only on the maxim through which you can at the same time will that it should become a universal law'.

CHAPTER

3

What critical ethics can achieve

'The opposite of a correct statement is a false statement, but the opposite of a profound truth may be another profound truth.'[1]

Learning outcomes

After reading this chapter, you should be able to:
- Understand the meaning of cognitivism.
- Understand the meaning of non-cognitivism.
- Evaluate the suggested methodology for rational argument within a non-cognitivist framework.

3.1 CAN ETHICAL POSITIONS BE PROVED?

Before examining the application of consequentialist and deontological approaches to ethical issues in health care, it is worth examining in more detail a point raised in Chapter 1. There we argued that a knowledge of the ethical codes governing practice was not sufficient for the solution of all the ethical problems encountered in health care. A critical ethical approach was needed which would examine the principles that were being implicitly or explicitly used in ethical discussions and consider what justification could be given for them. This claim might be taken to imply that it is possible to prove that certain ethical standards are correct and others are wrong in the sense that the flat earth theory would now generally be considered to be wrong. However, the adoption of a critical ethical approach to these issues does not assume that certain ethical positions are capable of being proved to be right and that others can be shown to be wrong. Some ethical theories do incorporate this claim but others do not.

It might be argued at this point that if an ethical theory does not prove that one position is right and another wrong then there is no point in adopting a critical ethical approach. After all, if it is just a matter of opinion which position is right, why do we need to examine these different theories? If it is ultimately up to us to decide what is right and this is quite compatible with someone else disagreeing, why do we need to consider the different philosophical theories that can be applied to ethical issues in health care?

3.2 COGNITIVISM VERSUS NON-COGNITIVISM

The labels for the two different views outlined above are cognitivism and non-cognitivism. These views cut across the distinction between consequentialist and deontological theories since both of these theories can be combined with either cognitivism or non-cognitivism. Stated formally, cognitivism is the view that moral judgements are statements that are capable of being true or false. So just as it is true or false that you are sitting in a library reading this book or that you are 35 years old, similarly, moral claims about what ought to be done are capable of being shown to be true or false.

Non-cognitivism is just the denial of the claim that moral judgements are statements capable of being true or false. This denial can be combined with a number of different positive views about the status of moral claims. These range from claiming that moral judgements are expressions of emotion[2,3] to claiming that they indicate ultimate preferences that we wish to adopt.[4,5] For example, we might think that life is something that is valuable even if the individual is not conscious. This is a position that we wish to adopt which is indicative of a fundamental attitude. Someone else might adopt a different view arguing that only life that is capable of supporting consciousness is valuable. Therefore, according to a non-cognitivist account it is possible for there to be ultimate disagreement between people who hold different ultimate preferences or express different emotions towards ethical issues.

Mill presented his consequentialist theory as a cognitivist theory since he believed that it was possible to prove the fundamental principle of morality that he called the Greatest Happiness Principle (see 2.2.3). However, both Singer[6] and Hare[7] adopt non-cognitivist approaches believing that it is possible for there to be disagreement between fundamental ethical positions.

Although there have been accounts recently that support a cognitivist approach[8], many consider that a non-cognitivist account is correct and that it is possible for there to be disagreement about what is right or wrong in moral questions. If you consider this to be correct, then it might appear that there is no future in undertaking a critical ethical approach to ethical issues in health care if ultimately it is up to each individual to decide what is right. If these views just reflect an individual's subjective preferences and subjective preferences differ, why embark on this sort of discussion? Indeed, what scope is there for rational discussion about ethical problems if ultimately it is up to the individual to decide what ought or ought not to be done?

3.3 RATIONAL DISCUSSION WITHIN A NON-COGNITIVIST FRAMEWORK

If a non-cognitivist view is adopted, there is still scope for the sort of rational discussion incorporated in critical ethics. We illustrate this using examples of abortion and embryo research to indicate the sort of procedure that would be employed in a critical ethical approach.

3.3.1 Isolation of principles

The first step in such a discussion is to find out what principles someone is using to justify their position.

ABORTION EXAMPLE

For example, if someone holds that all elective abortions are wrong we could enquire what principle they were using to support this position. This blanket condemnation of abortion with no qualifications for, for example, pregnancies commenced as a result of rape, might be supported by appealing to the sanctity of human life. Human life has intrinsic value and it is wrong to terminate something that has intrinsic value.

3.3.2 What do the principles mean?

Having ascertained the nature of the principle that is being used to justify the ethical position that has been taken about abortion, the second step in the discussion is to seek a greater understanding of what this principle means. Why is the principle limited to human life? At this point, the supporter of the original view about abortion might claim that the principle is just an example of the wider principle that all life forms are sacred. One would then need to know what it is about life itself that makes it intrinsically valuable. Does this principle extend to plant life as well as animal life? If the principle is being restricted to human life, what makes human life valuable as opposed to the lives of other species?

We would also need to know exactly what constitutes life. When is life supposed to have begun and what counts as the end of life? In the case of abortion, is life counted as having begun at conception? Answers to these sorts of questions would provide a far greater understanding of the view that is being held. They might even occasion a change in the original view once a fuller awareness of the exact meaning of the principle that was being used was gained.

3.3.3 What are the implications of these principles?

A change in an original view taken by someone might also result from the third step which could be taken in a critical ethical discussion. Having gained a fuller understanding of precisely what the principle one is appealing to means, changes of view could result when the implications of adopting this principle are pointed out. If we remain with the issue of abortion, the view might be held that abortions are justified if the fetus is discovered to be suffering from Down's syndrome. One principle that might be appealed to in justification of this position is that the quality of life of an individual suffering from Down's syndrome and the impact on the quality of life of those individuals who will be living with and caring for this individual is such that a termination is justified. However, if this justification is advanced, then one implication of this is that, if the presence of Down's syndrome has not been detected in the fetus, but the baby that is born is suffering from Down's syndrome, then the infanticide will be perfectly justified on the basis of the principle that was used to justify an abortion in these sorts of cases. Indeed, in the UK, since screening for Down's syndrome is only offered routinely to women over 35, most Down's syndrome children are born to mothers under 35 since they have not been screened during pregnancy. It might therefore be thought perfectly justifiable to accept the implications of this principle and hence the justifiability of infanticide in the case of these babies.

3.3.4 Change or qualification of original principles

However, holders of the original position with respect to abortions might not be prepared to accept the implication that the principle they are adopting would lead to the justification of infanticide. If they are not, then a fourth step in critical ethical discussion could come into play. They will either have to change their original view about the justifiability of abortions in these sorts of cases or appeal to a different principle to justify their original view. If they wish to qualify the principle that they used in the original justification of their views about abortion they might draw a distinction between a fetus and a baby. They might argue that their original principle only justified the termination of life in fetuses and did not apply to babies. The question they would then have to address is what are they taking to be the morally significant difference between a baby and a fetus? Why should one suppose that there is a moral difference between the two? Why is the location of the individual considered to be morally relevant? Is it justifiable to treat the premature baby differently from the fetus at the same stage of development? Answers to these questions might well lead again either to a modification of the original position or a change in the principle to which appeal is made. The basic demand that they are having to satisfy is that of consistency between the principles that they hold and the implications of these principles in cases other than the one under consideration.

EMBRYO RESEARCH EXAMPLE

Another example of this stage of discussion at work is apparent when we consider how the principle of the sanctity of human life might be invoked in the area of embryo research. Someone might hold the view that embryo research even only up to 14 days is wrong. The principle to which appeal is made to support this position might very well be the principle of the sanctity of human life. However, it might be pointed out in reply to this justification that at this stage of development we do not have a specific individual who could be said to have a right to life. At this stage, one fertilised egg might evolve into two individuals, two eggs into one individual or no individuals might evolve at all but instead a tumour rather than a fetus might result.

At this point the individual might well modify his or her original position and argue that what is sacrosanct is the potential for human life. Their rejection then of research on embryos would be based not on the sanctity of life of the embryo itself but in terms of its potential to become a human life and it is this that it is sacrosanct. Having modified the principle in this way, we can now appeal to the third step in critical ethical discussion (see 3.3.3) and consider the implications of this new principle that is being advocated. Presumably, sperm and eggs have the same potential as an embryo for developing into an individual and so this would mean that this new principle would arguably generate the judgement that all forms of reproductive control are wrong. This might well be a position that someone holding this principle does not want to accept and if this is the case, either the principle will have to be modified or rejected in favour of one that does not have this implication.

Therefore, although it might be accepted that fundamental moral principles are ultimately not susceptible to proof, this still leaves a very wide scope for the use of critical ethical discussion. Indeed, when this discussion has been undertaken, there might well be less disagreement over ultimate principles than has previously been the case. There is still much that can be done by the use of a critical ethical approach even if one adopts a non-cognitivist position where moral judgements are not taken to be statements that are capable of being shown to be true or false.

3.4 SINGER'S VIEW SUBJECTED TO CRITICAL ETHICAL DISCUSSION

The outline of the scope of critical ethical discussion that has been given can be illustrated in detail by taking an example of a non-cognitivist view and subjecting it to the sort of discussion just described. The example that I take is from Peter Singer's book, *Practical Ethics*[6].

Singer advocates a non-cognitivist consequentialist view which claims that actions are right in proportion as they maximise the satisfaction of the interests of those affected in a situation[9]. This is clearly a consequentialist view since the value of actions lies in their consequences and what has intrinsic value is the satisfaction of interests. On the face of it, this seems an attractive view and one which many might readily accept but, as we shall see, a closer examination reveals it to be quite controversial.

3.4.1 Isolation of Singer's principle

Singer proposes that when considering a moral problem we should give equal consideration to the interests of all those affected. Interests should be treated equally regardless of who possesses them. They are to be weighed to seek the maximum satisfaction of interests and no priority can be given to one interest over another simply by virtue of who happens to have it. It is the interests themselves that are weighed, and an interest cannot have more weight merely because it is possessed by you or someone you know.

3.4.2 What does this principle mean?

The controversial aspects of this proposal begin to become apparent when we enquire what sort of beings can be said to have interests. Having ascertained what principle Singer is advocating we now take the second step in the discussion and seeking a greater understanding of what this principle means. Without this critical ethical approach, we might have assumed without reflection that the principle only applies to human beings but, as we shall see, that would be to misunderstand Singer's position.

According to Singer, a necessary condition for a being to be able to possess an interest is that the being be sentient or conscious, that is, capable of feeling. A fundamental interest would be, for example, the interest we have in feeling pleasure and avoiding pain. Therefore, we can see that life itself is not sufficient for the possession of interests since there are life forms that are not conscious. For example, plants are living but they do not have a central nervous system that would allow them to be capable of feeling.

What about fetuses? Can fetuses be said to possess interests? Singer argues that until about the eighteenth week, the fetus has an insufficiently developed nervous system to be capable of feeling and hence to be capable of having interests. Therefore, although the pre-18–week fetus is alive, it does not have interests and hence an implication of the acceptance of Singer's principle is that in moral dilemmas involving pre18–week fetuses, the fetus will have no interests to be entered into the calculation seeking the maximum satisfaction of interests.

I have stated the desire to feel pleasure and to avoid pain as being one of the fundamental interests that Singer has in mind. However, there are other more sophisticated interests than this and the question arises whether all sentient beings are capable of having all possible interests. An interest that is particularly relevant in the field of health care is the interest we have in the continuation of our lives. What characteristics must a conscious being have in order to be capable of this interest? According to Singer, the sentient being must be aware of his or her continued existence over time, that is, be self-conscious. It is only self-conscious beings that are capable of having an interest in the continuation of their lives.

Singer proposes to use the term 'person' to refer to conscious beings who are, in addition, rational and self-conscious. Rationality involves, at the very least, the ability to make simple plans of action although many 'persons' possess far more than this minimal level of rationality. It is important to remember precisely what Singer means by his definition of 'person' since this does not correspond in all respects with the usual usage of this word. He is stipulating a definition of this word and some of his subsequent claims sound very strange unless it is remembered precisely how he uses the word 'person'.

Following an argument put forward by Tooley[10], Singer continues his argument by claiming that one can only be said to possess a right to something if one is capable of having the corresponding interest. So, for example, one can only be said to have a right to life if one is capable of having an interest in one's life continuing and this interest can only be possessed by those beings that Singer labels 'persons'.

If we draw the strands of this position together, we see the following classifications emerging. The species *Homo sapiens* contains three different groups according to Singer's account. The first group comprises those beings that are living but not sentient, for example, the pre-eighteen week fetus and certain beings towards the end of life. The second group is those that are conscious but not self-conscious, for example, the post-18–week fetus, young infants and those that are just conscious towards the end of life. Finally, wehave those members of the species *Homo sapiens* are 'persons' who in Singer's sense of this term, and thiscovers the majority of adults and children beyond immediate infancy.

3.4.3 Implications of Singer's principle

This analysis of the meaning of the principle proposed by Singer reveals at the third stage of our critical ethical discussion some rather surprising implications which conflict with many commonly held views. For example, birth is often thought to mark a morally significant dividing line in the development of an individual. By morally significant, we mean it is often thought to justify a difference in treatment between the fetus and the baby. One implication of Singer's account will be to deny this view since both before and after birth one will be dealing with a being that is sentient but not a 'person'.

Another important implication of Singer's account is that it denies another commonly held belief that human life, meaning the lives of those members of the species *Homo sapiens*, is of more value than the lives of other species just by virtue of their membership of this species. Species other than *Homo sapiens* will also have sentient members and, indeed, some species will in addition be 'persons'. Chimpanzees are given as one such example based on the observations made by Jane

Goodall[11]. She observed evidence of chimpanzees making plans for future behaviour which is one sign of the possession of rationality and self-consciousness.

Singer's distinction, which cuts across the distinction between species, has some startling implications which were not evident in the original formulation of his principle but which have become apparent during this process of critical ethical discussion. One example of the implication of ceasing to regard membership of species as morally significant can be seen in the following. Let us assume, for the sake of argument, that a horse is just a sentient being and not a 'person'. There are situations when a horse breaks a leg, in which consideration of the interests of the horse will lead to the judgement that the life of the horse ought to be terminated. The amount of pain that the horse is in is the factor that determines that the horse ought to be put down.

Compare this situation with the way we treat members of our own species who are sentient but not self-conscious. If we take the case of a severely damaged new-born infant who, even with every available technical assistance, is only likely to live for three months, it is often argued that everything should be done to insure the maximum duration of this individual's life. The amount of pain is not given the same consideration as in the case of the horse because it is being taken to be morally significant that the baby is a member of the species *Homo sapiens*.

Even if this position is not taken, it is often thought to be morally preferable to follow what might be called the course of passive euthanasia where nursing care alone is administered and the infant is 'allowed to die'. However, if we adopt Singer's position and treat interests equally regardless of who possesses them then the pain of the horse, which is sentient, has to be considered in the same way as the pain of the new-born infant. If we think that the maximum satisfaction of interests is achieved if the horse is shot then it might well be the case that the maximum satisfaction of the interests of those affected will be achieved if a course of active euthanasia is adopted with the new-born infant.

3.4.4 Should Singer's principle be changed or qualified?

This critical ethical discussion of Singer's principle that we ought to seek for the maximum satisfaction of the interests involved in a situation reveals the complexity of this view, and just how much revision of ordinary implicitly held moral convictions would be necessary if we were to adopt his proposal. Of course, we might argue conversely that Singer's principle has to be changed since it conflicts with many strongly held moral convictions. The initial formulation of this principle at the start of our discussion might have led many people to accept it as sounding relatively innocuous and self-evident. However, this examination reveals how radical the proposal is. The critical ethical approach has therefore greatly advanced our understanding of this issue.

It is not to be assumed from this discussion that we should now accept Singer's views since we might argue that Singer needs to change his principle. For example, one could argue for the moral significance of the species *Homo sapiens* on the grounds that, unlike some other species, it is a species that can have 'persons' as its members. Alternatively, one could argue for the moral significance of the species *Homo sapiens* on religious grounds. What we hope has become apparent by this illustration using Singer's view is the advantage of subjecting ethical views to the sort of critical analysis outlined in this chapter. Even if a non-cognitivist view is accepted, a great deal can be done by rational discussion in the ways outlined.

LEARNING EXERCISES

1. Do you think that it is possible to prove that certain ethical views are correct?
2. 'It is right to shoot a horse who is in agony after breaking a leg but it is never right to kill human beings who are suffering even if they want to die. This is because the lives of human beings are more important than those of animals.' Critically assess this view.
3. If it is ultimately up to each individual to decide what is right, what scope, if any, does this leave for rational discussion about ethical questions?

REFERENCES

1. Bohr, N. 'My Father' in *Niels Bohr: His Life and Work*. Ed. S. Rosental (1982), Wiley, New York.
2. Stevenson, C.L. (1994) *Ethics and Language*. Yale University Press, USA.
3. Ayer, A.J. (1976) *Language, Truth and Logic*. Gollancz Press, London.
4. Hare, R.M. (1981) *Moral Thinking: Its levels, Method and Point*. Oxford University Press, Oxford.
5. Glover, J. (1977) *Causing Death and Saving Lives*. Penguin Books, London.
6. Singer, P. (1933) *Practical Ethics* (2nd edn). Cambridge University Press, Cambridge.
7. Hare, *op. cit.*
8. McNaughton, D. (1988) *Moral Vision: An Introduction to Ethics*. Blackwell, Oxford.
9. Singer, *op. cit.*, p13.
10. Tooley, M. (1983) *Abortion and Infanticide*. Clarendon Press, Oxford.
11. Goodall, J. (1971) *In the Shadow of Man*, Boston.

Key points
- Cognitivism. Moral judgements are statements capable of being true or false.
- Non-cognitivism. Moral judgements are not statements capable of being true or false. For example, they might be expressions of emotion or an ultimate preference that one has chosen to adopt.
- Four steps for a rational discussion within a non-cognitivist framework:
  1. Isolate principles.
  2. Examine the meaning of the principles.
  3. Consider the implications of the principles.
  4. Consider possible changes or qualifications to original principles.
- Embryo research. All research on human embryos is wrong because human life is sacred.
- The principle of equal consideration of interests. The interests of all those affected in a moral problem should be considered equally.
- Singer classifies human beings as living and non-sentient, sentient and 'persons'. 'Persons' are rational and self-conscious beings. Other species have members in each of these three categories. For example, some chimpanzees are 'persons' and so are some dolphins. Only beings who are either sentient or 'persons' can be said to have interests and no moral questions arise unless interests are affected.

CHAPTER 4

The Principle of Autonomy

'Those who expect to reap the blessings of freedom must, like men, undergo the fatigue of supporting it.'

Thomas Paine (1737–1809)

Learning outcomes

After reading this chapter, you should be able to:
- Understand the justification of the Principle of Autonomy from within a consequentialist framework.
- Understand the justification of the Principle of Autonomy from within a deontological framework.
- Be able to recognise when the Principle of Autonomy arises in ethical problems.
- Evaluate the different justifications that can be given for the Principle of Autonomy.

4.1 WHAT IS THE PRINCIPLE OF AUTONOMY?

In Chapter 1 we saw how a Principle of Autonomy is often appealed to, if only implicitly, in ethical debates. Let us consider another example now.

The multiple sclerosis example

Without consultation with the individual, a physician has instructed that a middle-aged woman who suffers frequent asthma attacks and has severe multiple sclerosis should not be resuscitated if she suffers a cardiac arrest during an asthma attack at the hospital. It is generally agreed that the quality of life of this individual is appalling but since she has not been consulted, what ought the nurses to do if she has a cardiac arrest? (Case study adapted from Beauchamp and Childress.)

The meaning of autonomy

In considering this question, a nurse might very well feel that the autonomy of the middle-aged woman has not been respected. What does this mean? Autonomy is, 'the capacity to think, decide, and act on the basis of such thought and decision freely and independently.' [2] The nurse presumably considers that the middle-aged woman has this capacity, that is, she is able to consider her case and make a decision about what she would like done in the event of a cardiac arrest.

The Principle of Autonomy

The thought that this woman's autonomy had not been respected indicates that the nurse considered that the Principle of Autonomy had not been respected by the physician. That is, that the physician had not respected the woman's right to be self-governing in this area, to think about and decide what she would like to happen in the event of a cardiac arrest.

Why should we accept such a Principle of Autonomy? If such a principle is adopted, should it always be adopted in preference to any other principle? Does the principle apply to all individuals or do the individuals in question have to possess a certain degree of rationality and maturity? Is it possible to renounce autonomy? What justification of this principle is given within consequentialist theories and deontological theories?

4.2 JUSTIFICATIONS OF THE PRINCIPLE OF AUTONOMY

Starting with this question first, I shall consider Mill's justification of the Principle of Autonomy and then the justification given by Kant.

4.2.1 Mill's justification of the Principle of Autonomy

As we have seen in Chapter 2, Mill put forward a hedonistic consequentialist or utilitarian theory stating that we ought to aim for the best outcomes. The best outcomes, according to Mill, are those that are productive of happiness. By happiness he meant, at least initially, pleasure and the absence of pain. Mill had views about how happiness might be achieved, and one of them was described in his essay, *On Liberty*, where he wrote:

> *'That the only purpose for which power can be rightfully exercised over any*
> *member of a civilized community, against his will, is to prevent harm to others.*
> *His own good, either physical or moral, is not a sufficient warrant. ... Over*
> *himself, over his own body and mind, the individual is sovereign.'* [3]

This Principle of Liberty, as Mill called it, could also be called a Principle of Autonomy. It advocates the sovereignty or self-rule of the individual over those aspects of his life that do not harm others. Even if we think that some course of action might be harmful to someone, we are not justified in intervening to prevent them acting in this way unless their action will harm others. Mill justifies this principle by claiming that its adoption of it lead to happiness, which is the only thing that possesses intrinsic value in Mill's system. Therefore, the Principle of Autonomy does not have its own independent justification but rather is justified by appeal to the Principle of Utility (see Chapter 2). Mill writes:

> *'It is proper to state that I forego any advantage which could be derived to my*
> *argument from the idea of abstract right as a thing independent of utility. I regard*
> *utility as the ultimate appeal on all ethical questions.'* [4]

Mill is therefore arguing for freedom from constraints over an individual's own actions when these do not harm others. This area of an individual's life should be subject to his autonomous control and comprises first, liberty of thought and feeling which includes the freedom to express and publish our thoughts. Second, we ought to have liberty to decide how to live our lives in the sense of having autonomous control over our choice of life plans. Lastly, we should have liberty to combine with others for a common purpose[5] (see 12.1.2, 12.1.3, 12.2, 15.3.2, 15.3.4, 15.4, 16.1, 16.2.1, 17.4).

On a first reading of this Principle of Autonomy, it would appear that Mill is advocating a highly libertarian position which would involve very few restrictions on an individual's control over his own life and actions. However, this impression is diminished when we subject the principle to a closer examination.

Range of application of the principle

The first question that needs to be settled is what is the range of application of this principle? Does it apply to all human beings? Mill excludes children and those who cannot look after themselves from the range of applicability. In such cases then, we might be justified in intervening in the lives of these individuals if we judge that certain of their actions are not good for them or if we think that they require protection. This qualification is clearly important when we consider health care decisions at the beginning and end of life when it would appear that the principle of autonomy does not have any direct application. It is also relevant when considering cases involving mental handicap, such as decisions about whether or not certain mentally handicapped individuals ought to be sterilised. Presumably, interference in the lives of individuals not covered by the principle of autonomy could not be regarded as an infringement of their autonomy since they are not deemed to be capable of autonomy.

It is clearly not enough for Mill to just exclude children as a class unless he has some way of determining when an individual ceases to be a child. All Mill says on this point is that individuals are children up to the age that the law recognises them to be adults. This, though, is clearly not adequate. Why should the law be deemed to be the judge of this point? After all, until comparatively recently, the law in the UK stated that an individual was a child until the age of 21 years; this has changed to 18 years and, in matters of medical and dental treatment, 16 years (see Family Law Reform Act 1969). Although recent legislation (Children Act 1989) obliges the courts and others to find out and act upon a child's wishes where possible, the important point is that the law should not be *assumed* to give the correct answers. The law might enshrine what is right but this cannot be assumed, as Mill did at this stage of his account.

What needs specification are the characteristics that an individual needs to possess in order to be able to exercise autonomy and these characteristics might vary depending on the decision involved. For example, it might be felt that a 14-year-old child was too young to take the decision to donate a kidney to his or her mother. Presumably, what is required is a certain level of ability that enables one to make plans, envisage ways of carrying out these plans, understand information provided and evaluate various alternatives that are proposed. What this requires in detail will depend on the complexity of the problem in question. Many mentally handicapped individuals have sufficient of these characteristics to enable them to exercise autonomy over many of the everyday decisions with which they are faced. However, they might not satisfy these criteria when a complex health care decision regarding them is required.

Therefore, a blanket exclusion or inclusion of certain individuals within the class of autonomous individuals is not appropriate. What is needed is a matching of the level of rationality and maturity that is required for the specific decision in question. The level of rationality and maturity required will depend on the complexity of the decision to be taken.

What is an 'other'?

The second question we can raise about Mill's Principle of Autonomy concerns what is to be understood as an 'other'. Mill considers that it is only justifiable to intervene in the life of an individual to prevent harm to others. What sort of beings is it possible to harm? For example, is the fetus to be regarded as a being that can be harmed by an action? If a mother took heroin during pregnancy, would this provide a justification for taking the baby into care by the local authority on the grounds that it had been harmed when a fetus?

If the fetus were to be regarded as an 'other' then this might make it justifiable to intervene in the life of the pregnant woman to, for example, prevent her smoking or drinking heavily. These would be life plans that she could no longer adopt on the grounds that they harmed another. Of course, it is important to notice two points here. Mill only argues that intervention is justifiable to prevent harm to others. He does not say that intervention ought always to take place, but only that this is the only justification for such intervention. Second, he does not specify what form that intervention ought to take. In other words, it must not be assumed to be legal intervention. There are, after all, many interventions that one makes in the lives of children that are not legal interventions.

If the fetus is not regarded as an 'other', but as just part of the woman's body, then the Principle of Autonomy would allow her, one would think, to adopt the lifestyle of drinking or smoking if she wished. Of course, Mill might argue that the adoption of such a lifestyle in this condition is indicative that the individual is not competent to exercise autonomy in this area of her life. Her lack of ability is indicated by the adoption of this particular life plan. However, if this argument is followed, the initial libertarian impression created by Mill's principle would be lost and instead it would be seen as highly restrictive of individual liberty.

How far do 'others' extend?

A third question that we should raise to understand the application of Mill's principle within the context of health care issues is how far do the 'others' extend when we are considering harm? If the behaviour of the individual described above caused her to develop lung cancer or to produce a baby that required the facilities of an intensive care unit, would this be harming others? After all, the cost of this care would reduce resources and might even deprive another individual of the care they needed if there were insufficient resources. Might it not also be said to be harming the relatives and friends of the individual who has adopted this life plan? Indeed, there might not be very many actions that we could choose to adopt which do not have some effect on others in this sort of sense.

Mill attempted to deal with this sort of objection when he wrote:

> '*When I say only himself, I mean directly and in the first instance; for whatever affects himself may affect others through himself.*' [6]

This, as it stands, is not very precise, and we would need some indication of when an effect ceases to be direct and becomes indirect. Depending on this interpretation will depend how restrictive or libertarian Mill's principle turns out to be.

Conflict with other principles

Finally, we need to consider what Mill would say about cases where the requirements of the Principle of Autonomy conflict with other principles that might be considered applicable in the situation. In the 'multiple sclerosis example', presumably the physician thought that the decision not to resuscitate would be for the benefit of the woman. He did not consult her to ascertain whether or not she would consider the course of action beneficial, but took the decision himself. He was therefore appealing to a Principle of Beneficence, the principle of doing what is viewed to be best for the individual. He has also treated this principle as overriding the Principle of Autonomy.

To take another example of this conflict of principles, we might consider the following case. An individual who is a Jehovah's Witness might refuse to have a blood transfusion in the knowledge that without it they are likely to die. This decision constitutes an expression of their autonomy but is in conflict with what is considered will promote the well-being of this individual, namely, continued life.

Now, although frequently Mill writes as though the Principle of Liberty has independent standing, consistency requires that it is justified by the fact that it is productive of utility. Mill considers that it will lead to an increase in what he calls utility in the largest sense;

> '... *grounded on the permanent interests of man as a progressive being. Those interests, I contend, authorize the subjection of individual spontaneity to external control only in respect to those actions of each which concern the interest of other people.*' [7]

Therefore, if there is a case where it is considered that more utility will be produced by overriding a person's autonomy, then this would be justified if we accept Mill's consequentialist justification of the Principle of Autonomy. Respecting the autonomy of individuals, within a consequentialist justification, is only valued to the extent that it will increase utility. When it does not, then the Principle of Autonomy will be overridden.

4.2.2 Kant's justification of the Principle of Autonomy

Kant formulates his Principle of Autonomy in the *Groundwork of the Metaphysic of Morals* in the following way:

> '*The Idea of the will of every rational being as a will which makes universal law.*' [8]

Kant, unlike Mill, is concentrating on autonomy of the will rather than autonomy of thought and action which are Mill's major concerns. Individuals, as rational beings, exercise their autonomy by originating universal laws. However, and this might seem like a limitation on our autonomy, we cannot make any subjective principle we like into a universal law. Only those subjective principles that pass the test of the categorical imperative (see 2.3.1) can become universal laws. The categorical imperative, though, is not some external constraint which limits our autonomy . Rather, it incorporates a requirement of rationality that one be able to universalise proposed subjective principles without this involving any form of contradiction.

This Principle of Autonomy is applicable to all rational beings in virtue of their rationality. Therefore, in exercising one's autonomy by originating universal laws one must recognise that other individuals have autonomy as well . Kant expresses this point by saying that we must treat other rational individuals as ends in themselves and not treat them as means to other ends. He writes:

> 'Act in such a way that you always treat humanity, whether in your own person
> or in the person of any other, never simply as a means but always at the same time
> as an end.' [9]

As rational agents, other people as well as ourselves can set ends and make rational choices. There must be mutual respect for each individual's autonomy.

One of the implications that Kant draws from what he calls 'the formula of the end in itself' is that suicide is wrong since the adoption of a principle allowing suicide would involve treating myself as a means rather than as an end. Kant writes:

> 'If he does away with himself in order to escape from a painful situation, he is
> making use of a person merely as a means to maintain a tolerable state of affairs
> till the end of his life.' [10]

Kant also uses this formula to show the wrongness of false promises:

> 'The man who has a mind to make a false promise to others will see at once that
> he is intending to make use of another man merely as a means to an end he does
> not share. For the man whom I seek to use for my own purposes by such a promise
> cannot possibly agree with my way of behaving to him, and so cannot share the
> end of the action.' [11]

So, in exercising one's autonomy, the principle which one adopts must conform to the requirements of rationality. One must be able to universalise the principle without there being any sort of contradiction. In addition, one must recognise that the content of possible principles is limited by the recognition that other individuals are also autonomous agents.

Unlike Mill, Kant is not arguing for the acceptance of the autonomy principle on the grounds that it will yield beneficial consequences. Acting on principles that can become universal laws is good in itself. It is this motivation that makes an action right and the consequences of an action neither add to nor subtract from the value of the action. To understand this point fully, it might be useful to consider an example. A decision is taken to offer a particular therapy to an individual on the grounds that on the evidence available it is the best treatment for this particular individual's condition. The principle that is being employed is that of doing one's best to help others in need of assistance. If the particular treatment turns out not to benefit the individual then that does not make the action of prescribing that treatment wrong. The principle that guided that action provided the justification for claiming that it was right. Conversely, if the treatment does benefit the individual, this does not make the action any more right than it was. It is the principle which motivated the action that makes it right.

In addition, it is important to note that it is only the motivation of acting on principles that can become universal laws that can give an action moral worth. Acting from other motives might be commendable or blameable but it is only acting from principles that can become universal laws that gives an action moral worth. It is acting from this motive that Kant calls acting from the motive of duty. To act from duty is to act on principles that can become universal laws (see 10.1, 12.1.2,12.2, 13.4, 15.3.2, 17.7).

The application of Kant's Principle of Autonomy, like that of Mill's, requires a certain level of rationality so that certain individuals who have impaired rationality will be excluded from the range of the principle. Clearly, an understanding of what it is to act on a principle and what is involved in universalising a principle is necessary to establish Kant's Principle of Autonomy as applicable to an individual.

4.3 APPLICATION OF THE PRINCIPLE OF AUTONOMY TO SOME EXAMPLES

These abstract accounts of how the Principle of Autonomy might be justified on consequentialist and deontological grounds can perhaps be better understood if we consider the application of some of these points to health care issues (see also 16.2.1).

Examples involving informed consent
One way in which the Kantian principle of respect for the autonomy of another individual might be ignored is if incomplete information is given to an individual about the alternative treatments that are available. It is, of course, no easy matter to determine what will count as complete information but certain cases present clear examples of where insufficient information has been given. Clearly, if the individual is not properly informed then his or her autonomy is limited since his or her consent to the treatment is not based on all the available information. Similarly, if the information is presented in such a way that the treatment that is preferred by the health carer is shown as being the 'right' choice, then this impairs the autonomy of the individual trying to decide whether or not to consent to this form of treatment. The carer is not treating the individual as a rational being, as an end in himself.

A consequentialist approach to this problem would consider different questions as relevant. Autonomy is only to be valued if it yields the best outcomes. It might well be the case that sometimes best outcomes are achieved when incomplete or biased information is provided so that the individual seeking treatment chooses what is regarded as the best treatment by the health care team.

Lying to benefit

Another way in which the Kantian respect for the autonomy of an individual might be ignored is if a health carer lies to an individual. If the health carer decides in a particular case to lie about a person's diagnosis, then this is to treat that individual as a means towards a particular end rather than an end in himself. It is to deny that individual's autonomy. This sort of case might arise when the health carer does not think that it would be beneficial for the individual to know the truth, but this sort of paternalistic intervention would not be justified if one accepts Kant's account.

Conversely, adopting Mill's justification of the Principle of Autonomy might lead to a different evaluation in this sort of case. This is because the consequences of not revealing the true diagnosis in this particular case might produce more happiness or less unhappiness than respecting autonomy.

Recognition of the values of an individual

Another example concentrates more on those aspects of autonomy that are highlighted by Mill. In the *International Council of Nurses Code for Nurses: Ethical Concepts Applied to Nursing* (see Appendix), there is a clause which states:

> 'The nurse, in providing care, promotes an environment in which the values,
> customs and spiritual beliefs of the individual are respected.' [12]

This explicitly recognises that region of autonomy that Mill discusses when he talks of our liberty to choose our own life plans, tastes and pursuits.

An example of the sort of case where this can become problematic is illustrated in the case of the Jehovah's Witness which we mentioned earlier. What does the health carer do if death without a blood transfusion is imminent? Does the health carer respect the person's values if the individual has refused consent to a blood transfusion, or ought the health carer to override this decision by, for example, obtaining a court order to go ahead with the transfusion? Presumably, Mill would advocate that we consider the effects of denying autonomy in an area which he considers is legitimately within the individual's control and compare that with the effects of allowing this life plan to be adopted with the consequent death of the individual.

4.4 WHICH JUSTIFICATION OF AUTONOMY IS TO BE PREFERRED?

In debating the merits of a consequentialist or deontological justification for the Principle of Autonomy, I should like to argue for the latter support although based on somewhat different grounds to those proposed by Kant. Autonomy of individuals is something that needs to be recognised irrespective of the consequences of such recognition and needs to be upheld even in cases where it is thought that the consequences will not be the best.

The reason for this is that the recognition of autonomy as having intrinsic value is essential for the survival of relationships which we have with other people (see 15.3.4). In contracting different relationships with people, we recognise that people cannot be exchanged and that individuals should not be used as a means towards some further end. They are properly, as Kant recognised, ends in themselves.

We all live within a system of relationships of which the relationship we have with members of a health care team which we choose to consult is just one example. In order for these relationships to survive we have to trust individuals to be true to their relationships, for example, to be a true friend, husband or colleague. If a friend communicates information to someone else that they were told in confidence, we talk about them betraying the trust we had in them as a friend. Similarly, when we consult a member of a health care team, we trust that individual to be true to the relationship that they have formed with us. At a minimum level, this will involve communicating truthfully and fully when requested to do so. It will also involve the recognition that the individual is an active member of the health care team and is in the majority of cases, the one who is responsible for the final decision that is taken about treatment or whatever else concerns the individual. For there to be relationships like this the autonomy of all the parties to the relationship must be recognised. In the case of the Jehovah's Witness, although the death of the individual without a blood transfusion might be counted as a harm by other members of the health care team, it must be recognised that this is not viewed as a harm for the individual who is the Jehovah's Witness. To be true to their relationships in these sort of cases, the autonomy of the individual must be recognised.

LEARNING EXERCISES

1. Should members of health care teams always tell the truth to individuals who consult them? Consider this question from within a consequentialist framework and from within a deontological framework.
2. What characteristics must an individual possess for the Principle of Autonomy to be applicable?

REFERENCES

1. Beauchamp, T.L. and Childress, J.F. (1983) *Principles of Biomedical Ethics* (2nd edn). Oxford University Press, Oxford, p304.
2. Gillon, R. (1990) *Philosophical Medical Ethics*. John Wiley, Chichester, UK, p60.
3. Mill, J.S. 'On Liberty'. In G. Himmelfarb (ed.) (1985) *On Liberty* . Penguin Books, London, p68.
4. *Ibid*, pp69–70.
5. *Ibid*, p71.
6. *Ibid*, p71.
7. *Ibid*, p70.
8. Kant, I. (1948) 'Groundwork of the Metaphysic of Morals'. In H.J.Paton (ed) (1948) *The Moral Law*. Hutchinson University Library, London, p93.
9. *Ibid*, p91.
10. *Ibid*, p91.
11. *Ibid*, p92.
12. *International Council of Nurses Code for Nurses: Ethical Concepts Applied to Nursing.*

Key points
- The Principle of Autonomy. In certain areas an individual has a right to be self-governing.
- Mill's Harm Principle. The only justification for exercising power over an individual is to prevent that individual harming others.
- Who are others and how far does this extend?
- Autonomy can be overridden if more utility will be produced by doing this.
- Kant's Principle of Autonomy. 'The idea of the will of every rational being as a will which makes universal law.' [8]
- Informed consent and the Principle of Autonomy.
- Lying to benefit and the Principle of Autonomy.
- Recognition of the values of an individual and the Principle of Autonomy.

CHAPTER 5

The Principles of Beneficence and Non-maleficence

'Primum non nocere; above all ... do no harm'.

—A fundamental medical principle (from the Hippocratic Oath; see Appendix B.)

Learning outcomes

After reading this chapter, you should be able to:
- Understand the meanings of the Principles of Beneficence and Non-maleficence.
- Evaluate the relative merits of a consequentialist and deontological justification of the Principles of Beneficence and Non-maleficence.
- Appreciate some of the difficulties with assessing benefits and harms.
- Appreciate in ethical problems where there might be supposed to be a conflict between the requirements of the Principle of Autonomy on the one hand and the Principles of Beneficence and Non-maleficence on the other.

5.1 WHAT ARE THE PRINCIPLES OF BENEFICENCE AND NON-MALEFICENCE?

As we have seen in earlier examples, the Principle of Autonomy is not the only principle appealed to in health care decisions. Appeals are also made to the Principles of Beneficence and Non-maleficence (see 12.1.2, 15.3.1, 15.3.2, 15.3.3). The following example provides an illustration of all these principles at work.

The new drug example

There is a new drug which should give an excellent chance of remission for an individual who has leukaemia. However, this drug has not yet been evaluated over the long term so that there might be the risk of, as yet unknown, harmful side-effects. The consultant considers that the new drug should be prescribed. Discussion about the possibility of risks should be omitted on the grounds that the individual would not have sufficient medical competence to evaluate the these. The consultant is in the best position to determine which treatment is best for the individual. The nurse considers that the treatment options should be fully discussed with the individual and that the individual has the right to decide on the treatment.

The consultant is appealing to the Principle of Beneficence since the assumption is that the new drug will be for the benefit or well-being of the individual. The consultant also appreciates the relevance of the Principle of Non-maleficence, one ought to do no harm, since the risk of possible harmful side-effects has been considered. The nurse is giving priority to the Principle of Autonomy since this is considered to be an area in which the individual has the right to be self-governing. The individual has the right to be given sufficient information about the possible available treatments and then to decide which treatment to have.

5.2 JUSTIFICATIONS OF THE PRINCIPLES OF BENEFICENCE AND NON-MALEFICENCE

As with the Principle of Autonomy, we need to consider how the Principles of Beneficence and Non-maleficence could be justified in consequentialist and deontological terms (see12.3, 13.2, 13.3, 15.3, 15.4, 16.2, 17.4).

5.2.1 Consequentialist justification
ONLY ONE PRINCIPLE?
It might be argued that really we have only one principle here and that promoting well-being and not harming just represent opposite ends of a continuum. This is the position usually adopted by those who justify these principles in consequentialist terms (see13.2). Also, the Hippocratic Oath lists them together:

> *'I will use treatment to help the sick according to my ability and judgment, but I will never use it to injure or wrong them.'* (See Appendix.)

The reason for saying that these two principles might represent two ends of a continuum becomes apparent if one starts to ask what promoting benefit involves. If one adopts a hedonistic consequentialist position such as that advocated by Mill, then promoting benefit will involve seeking to maximise as much happiness as possible. Singer's view is that promoting benefit involves maximising interest satisfaction. We ought to perform positive acts to *promote* what is taken to be of benefit.

However, in addition to acts such as these which quite obviously fall under the Principle of Beneficence, we also have acts which could be said to be promoting benefit by removing unhappiness or states of affairs where interests are not satisfied. Possibly, the majority of health interventions are of this nature since they are attempting to *remove* a cause of unhappiness and in this way conform to the Principle of Beneficence. Treatments are designed to benefit an individual by curing a condition that was detracting from the well-being of that individual.

Thirdly, we have those acts, which could also be said to fall under the Principle of Beneficence, that are designed to promote well-being by *preventing* harm. Advances in preventative medicine provide a clear illustration of this, of which an obvious example is the immunisation programme.

From preventing harm, it is argued, it is a short step to the Principle of Non-maleficence which advocates that we ought not to inflict harm. We are benefiting individuals by not harming them. Indeed, Mill when he formulates his Principle of Utility (see 2.2.3), describes happiness as pleasure *and* the absence of pain.

One argument that one might advance to deny that there is a continuum between the Principle of Beneficence and the Principle of Non-maleficence is that the range of application of the two principles is different. The latter principle applies to everyone unlike the former principle. We do not have a duty to benefit everyone although we have a duty not to harm anyone.

However, this is precisely the point that consequentialist theories deny. They consider that we have a duty to produce as much good as possible and therefore that the range of application of the principles is equally wide. Just as it would be wrong to do harm to someone by, for example, murdering them, similarly, we have a duty to do much more good in the world than is currently the case. For example, in not giving more to charity, we are actually allowing many people to die and this is just as bad as killing someone. We are, after all, evaluating the rightness or wrongness of our actions by the consequences of our actions and consequences can be produced by omissions as well as acts.

Jonathan Glover is one who supports this sort of view, but he tempers it by suggesting that we have to work out priorities in our life. He writes:

> *The moral approach advocated here does not commit us, absurdly, to remedying all the evil in the world. It does not even commit us to spending our whole time trying to save lives. What we should do is work out what things are most important and then try to see where we ourselves have a contribution to make.'* [1]

This sort of position is examined in Chapter 7, when we look at the acts and omissions doctrine.

If we assume for the moment that we *can* make a distinction between positive actions and omissions, then we could list the *acts* of doing good, removing harm and preventing harm as being appropriate to the domain of beneficence leaving only the duty of not inflicting harm (*omission*) within the province of the Principle of Non-maleficence.

5.2.2 Deontological justification

Understood in this way, it is argued by supporters of deontological theories that there is an important difference between the Principle of Beneficence and the Principle of Non-maleficence. Kant, for example, talks of the duty of non-maleficence as being a *perfect duty* and the duty of beneficence as an *imperfect duty.*

Kant defines a perfect duty as 'one which allows no exception in the interest of inclination'.[2] What he means by this can be illustrated by the suicide example that was used in Chapter 4. Since the duty of non-maleficence, not inflicting harm, is a positive duty, then even if we have a strong inclination to end our lives, this does not entitle us to commit suicide and make an exception to the Principle of Non-maleficence. However, in the case of imperfect duties, such as the Principle of Beneficence, we can consult our inclinations in the sense that it is up to us to a certain extent to decide whom to help. If a doctor or nurse wishes to help care for the orphans in Rumania, he or she is not condemned on the grounds that, for example, there is more need in Iraq. There is some latitude to decide whom one will help but the duty not to inflict harm is applicable universally.

This distinction reflects a fairly widespread common sense intuition that perfect duties such as the duty of non-maleficence have greater stringency than imperfect duties. That is, our duty not to harm is greater than our duty to benefit. Therefore, in cases of conflict between beneficence and non-maleficence, non-maleficence will normally override beneficence. Let us take a somewhat frivolous example. There is one individual who could donate two of his organs to two other individuals and thereby save their lives at the expense of his own. The duty of not inflicting harm on this individual to benefit the other two will take precedence here. Interestingly, some consequentialists might have to reach a different decision since the consequences of two lives saved as opposed to one might appear to make the action of removing the organs the right action.

5.3 DESCRIPTION OF CASES

Although common sense intuition might draw this sort of distinction between the Principle of Beneficence and the Principle of Non-maleficence, there is a problem in some cases to decide which principle is applicable.

For example, consider a case[3] where a man has agreed to undergo tests with a view to donating bone marrow. The tests reveal the compatibility of the bone marrow. The individual then changes his mind about going ahead with the donation. How would we describe this case? What duty does the donor owe to the potential recipient of the bone marrow? Is it a duty of beneficence since it will remove harm, or is it to be described as falling under the Principle of Non-maleficence since deciding not to give bone marrow after having previously agreed to is to inflict harm? If deontological theories are correct then this will make a difference. If it is described as a duty of beneficence then this does not have the stringency of the duty of non-maleficence. The potential donor would not be obliged to go ahead with the donation. For consequentialists, the description of the action would presumably not make a difference to whether or not the action was obligatory . The consequences would be the same regardless of the description and actions are evaluated as being right or wrong depending on their consequences.

Another area where the description of the action might determine whether or not the case is deemed to fall under the Principle of Beneficence or the Principle of Non-maleficence is in the field of abortion. If we assume that we have an individual from the moment of conception whom it is possible to harm (see 3.4.2), what duty do we owe to this individual? Do we say that we owe him or her a duty of non-maleficence and thus that an abortion would be wrong since we are harming the fetus by killing it? Or do we say that the Principle of Beneficence allows us the latitude to decide whom we benefit and we are not obliged to benefit this particular individual?[4] Although we have a duty to benefit, we do not have a duty to benefit anyone in particular and when we decide to benefit a particular individual this is more accurately described as a case of supererogation, beyond the call of duty.

Of course, in the area of health care it might be argued that by becoming a health care professional one has taken on a duty to benefit the individuals who consult you. However, this is still a limitation on the range of application of the Principle of Beneficence since this duty is not owed to everyone.

5.4 ASSESSMENT OF BENEFITS AND HARMS

A major problem with the application of the Principles of Beneficence and Non-maleficence concerns how benefits and harms are to be assessed. What is to count as well-being , what is to count as harm and whose concept of harm and benefit are we to consider? The health care team's concept of what counts as a harm or benefit might well differ from the view held by the individual who is subject to their care.

It is important when considering this range of problems to recognise that well-being and harm are evaluative terms. Harms and benefits are not things that can objectively be determined to be present. They are not like determining how many people are in a room or whether a light is switched on or not. Rather, they depend on an individual's evaluation of the situation. Infliction of death, which might be viewed as the ultimate harm for an individual, might be viewed by some people in some situations as a benefit. Serious requests for euthanasia indicate that the individual's evaluation of their own life leads them to view death as a benefit rather than a harm.

In a less extreme case, a surgical procedure to amputate a hand might be considered, since the alternative of trying to save it will incur great pain and will also put the rest of the arm at risk. In terms of probabilities of success indicated by similar cases in the past, the best course of action will be to amputate the hand. However, what is needed is the individual's own assessment of what these alternatives mean to his life. A concert pianist might well think it worth the risk of trying to avoid amputation because of his or her lifestyle. This case illustrates two points. First, that benefits and harms need to be weighed against each other. Second, that the conclusion reached as a result of this weighing might well differ from individual to individual depending on how they view what counts as well-being for them.

5.5 THE PRINCIPLE OF AUTONOMY AND THE PRINCIPLE OF BENEFICENCE

This last point highlights the problem of what is to be done when there is a conflict between the health care team's weighing of benefits and harms and the individual's weighing of benefits and harms (see 16.2.1 and 16.2.3). In the 'new drug example' we saw that the consultant has weighed the benefits and harms of the different treatments. This would be described as *paternalistic*, since it is the health carer's evaluation of what would benefit the individual. Literally, the health carer is acting like a father by doing what he or she considers best for the individual and by assuming that it is appropriate to take some of these decisions for that individual. In this case the individual was not consulted about the treatment options. However, there are cases where the individual is consulted and their evaluation of benefits and harms differs from that of the health carers. Ought the individual's evaluation to be given priority always or is paternalistic intervention justified in some cases? In other words, what do we say about cases where the Principle of Beneficence appears to dictate one course of action, but this prescription would conflict with the requirements of the Principle of Autonomy?

The view that we advocate is that autonomy ought always to override these other principles, but that the difficult question to decide is whether or not the individual can be regarded as autonomous in each individual case. As we argued in Chapter 4, the characteristics necessary for autonomy will vary depending on the complexity of the decision required, but this still leaves latitude for differences of opinion about whether or not the Principle of Autonomy applies in an individual case.

For example, if someone adopts a life plan which we think is not the sort of life plan that a rational individual would adopt are we justified in denying that that individual has autonomy? In other respects, the individual might be exhibiting rationality in pursuance of this life plan. An individual might be choosing appropriate means to achieve the end that he or she has adopted, and their adherence to this end might be consistent with other aspects of their life. In other words, they would be exhibiting two characteristics that indicate rationality, but it is being judged that the life plan they have adopted makes it appropriate to deny that the Principle of Autonomy applies in this particular case. One such example is given by Beauchamp and Childress[5] where an individual is admitted to a mental institution on the grounds that the life plan they have adopted involves self-mutilation. Their belief in God has led them to think that God requires these sacrifices from them in order to prevent even greater harm to the rest of humanity.

The danger of allowing paternalistic evaluation of life plans is that this would enable one to deny that the individual is capable of an autonomous decision. This would therefore allow the possibility of a justified paternalistic intervention. Of course, if the Principle of Autonomy genuinely does not apply, then a paternalistic intervention justified by the Principle of Beneficence might well be appropriate. The justification would be that the individual being treated is unable to judge themselves in the particular case what would benefit them. So paternalism here is not being advocated in opposition to recognising autonomy because it is assumed that the Principle of Autonomy is not applicable. Where the Principle of Autonomy is applicable, then this should have precedence.

The Principle of Autonomy justifiably overrides the Principle of Beneficence and, indeed, the Principle of Non-maleficence for the following reason. If an individual has the characteristics necessary to exercise autonomy in a particular case then this implies the ability to judge what is beneficial or harmful for that individual. Given that we have argued that well-being and harm are evaluative terms, the evaluation of an individual who is capable of making an assessment of what constitutes well-being or harm for them ought to be the final court of appeal. This is justified on both deontological and consequentialist grounds. The latter justification would consist of arguing that the consequences were the best if this were advocated, since the determination of what counts as a good outcome has been made by the individual concerned. A deontological justification consists of pointing to the intrinsic worth of exercising autonomy (see 4.2.2)

This last point highlights that we only have the potential for conflict between the Principle of Beneficence and the Principle of Autonomy if we combine the Principle of Beneficence with a paternalistic evaluation of benefits and harms. If the individual's evaluation of benefits and harms is coupled with the Principle of Beneficence, then this is in conformity with the Principle of Autonomy. The individual will decide to do what he or she considers will be of most benefit to him or her.

LEARNING EXERCISES

1. Are the Principles of Beneficence and Non-maleficence totally distinct or are they just at different ends of a continuum? Give an example of an ethical dilemma in health care where the answer to this question would lead to different evaluations.
2. Can the Principle of Beneficence ever conflict with the Principle of Autonomy?

REFERENCES

1. Glover, J. (1982) *Causing Death and Saving Lives*. Penguin Books, London, p105.
2. Kant, I. 'Groundwork of the Metaphysic of Morals'. In H.J. Paton (ed) (1948) *The Moral Law*. Hutchinson University Library, London, p85.
3. Beauchamp, T.L. and Childress, J.F. (1983) *Principles of Biomedical Ethics* (2nd edn). Oxford University Press, Oxford, pp315–16.
4. Jarvis Thomson, J. (1986) 'A Defence of Abortion'. In P. Singer (ed.) *Applied Ethics*. Oxford University Press, Oxford, pp37–56.
5. Beauchamp and Childress, *op. cit.*, pp295–6.

Key points

- The Principles of Beneficence. The well-being or benefit of the individual ought to be promoted.
- The Principle of Non-maleficence. One ought to do no harm.
- Consequentialist justification of the Principles of Beneficence and Non-maleficence. Are they really at either end of a continuum from :
  1. promoting benefit, to
  2. removing harm, to
  3. preventing harm, to
  4. not inflicting harm?
- Ought we to spend our whole time remedying evil?
- According to deontological theories, the duty of non-maleficence is a perfect duty which allows for no exceptions.
- According to deontological theories, the duty of beneficence is an imperfect duty where we can consult our inclinations about who we shall benefit.
- What is to count as benefit and harm, and who should make the assessment?
- Does the Principle of Beneficence conflict with the Principle of Autonomy?

The Principle of Justice

'Into the discussion of human affairs, the questions of justice enters only where the pressure of necessity is equal, and that the powerful exact what they can, and the weak grant what they must.'

Thucydides (471–401 BC)

Learning outcomes

After reading this chapter, you should be able to:
- Understand consequentialist interpretations of the Principle of Justice.
- Evaluate whether or not consequentialist justifications of justice result in just treatment between individuals.
- Understand and evaluate Quality Adjusted Life Year (QALY) approaches as a basis for allocating health care resources.
- Understand the deontological interpretation of the Principle of Justice given by Rawls.

6.1 WHAT IS THE PRINCIPLE OF JUSTICE?

In Chapters 4 and 5, we concentrated on principles that have their central application within the sphere of the care of the individual. Now we shall be looking at a principle which is used in health care decisions which go beyond the particular individual. The Principle of Justice , that equals ought to be considered equally[1],is applicable in two areas of health care decisions. First, to decide what treatments should be made available within allocated resources. Second, who should receive treatments if there are not enough available for those who need them (see 15.3.1, 15.4, 17.4)? If a particular course of treatment is the most beneficial for that individual, it does not follow that the individual will be able to receive that treatment given limited resources. A principle of justice needs to be designed to provide a just way of distributing benefits between individuals.

The following example provides an illustration of the relevance of the Principle of Justice in allocating resources between individuals.

The artificial hip example

There are two individuals both of whom require an artificial hip. One is in her mid-20s and at the start of a promising medical career. The other is in her late 60s and retired. There are only enough resources for one hip replacement from within the current budget. If we apply the Principle of Justice, that equals ought to be considered equally, which of these individuals ought to receive the transplant?

To try to answer this question we need to gain a clearer understanding of precisely what the Principle of Justice means and how it might be justified.

6.2 CONSEQUENTIALIST INTERPRETATIONS OF JUSTICE

A distinction is drawn between the formal principle of justice, that equals ought to be considered equally, and various ways in which this might be interpreted. The formal principle is almost universally accepted and, as it stands, appears to be intuitively acceptable. Unfortunately, this formal principle is compatible with many different interpretations and it is these latter over which there is disagreement. Some of these interpretations lead to substantial principles that many might consider to be blatantly 'unjust'. We shall argue that one of these is incorporated in the consequentialist interpretation of a Principle of Justice.

Consequentialists, as we have seen, consider that what is of value is that the best outcome be produced and that actions or rules are right in proportion as they produce the best outcome. When it comes to considering a consequentialist justification of justice, Mill writes:

> '... *"everybody to count for one, nobody for more than one" might be written under the principle of utility as an explanatory commentary'.* [2]

He explains that what he means by this is that:

> '... *equal amounts of happiness are equally desirable, whether felt by the same or different people'.* [3]

What we can see from this is that the 'equals' referred to in Aristotle's formal Principle of Justice is not being taken to apply to individuals but instead to amounts of happiness. Therefore, although the first quotation gives the appearance of supporting equality between individuals, the explanatory comment makes it clear that what is intended is equality between amounts of happiness and not between individuals.

6.2.1 The consequentialist conception of justice ignores individuals

Now, what one would expect from a principle of distributive justice is that the principle would ensure an equitable distribution of benefits and burdens within society. However, Mill's interpretation of justice has not ensured this at all. If justice is to consist in equal amounts of pleasure being equally desirable then this claim is compatible with a very unfair distribution of happiness between individuals. The ultimate aim is the achievement of the greatest amount of happiness and equal amounts of happiness are equally desirable. Therefore, if the same amount is available to those who are well off as to those who are not so fortunate, this Principle of Justice says nothing about giving the benefit to the less advantaged individual. In other words, the achievement of the greatest amount of happiness is compatible with a very unequal distribution of that happiness between individuals.

Singer, another consequentialist whose theory we have discussed, will also be faced with the same difficulty as Mill. According to Singer, the best outcome consists in the maximum satisfaction of interests of those affected. To achieve this situation one must adopt the following principle:

> *'The essence of the principle of equal consideration of interests is that we give equal weight in our moral deliberations to the like interests of all those affected by our actions.'* [4]

In other words, his Principle of Justice is guaranteeing that interests be treated equally. It is not advocating that individuals be treated equally. From this it does not follow that there will be a just distribution of interest satisfaction over those affected. Similar interests are to be considered equally regardless of who possesses them, but this could lead to a very unequal distribution of interest satisfaction over the population.

6.2.2 The Principle of Declining Marginal Utility

Consequentialists usually make either or both of the following replies to this criticism. One reply consists in denying that the sort of situation that I have described will occur since they support the Principle of Declining Marginal Utility. This states that

> *'...for a given individual, a set amount of something is more useful when that individual has little of it than when he has a lot'.* [5]

For example, £5 given to a beggar is more useful that £5 given to a millionaire.

This principle translated into Singer's system is presumably as follows. The satisfaction of like interests by those who have more of their interests satisfied compared with those who have few of their interests satisfied will count for less interest satisfaction. In this way, they will guarantee a fair distribution of interest satisfaction between individuals.

However, the factual claim incorporated in the Principle of Declining Marginal Utility about how interest satisfaction will be achieved does not invalidate the point made above. Consequentialists cannot guarantee that outcomes will only be as good as possible when there is a fair distribution between individuals. The essence of their problem is that good outcomes are viewed as the maximum satisfaction of interests or pleasure and this is considered as a totality, divorced from individuals. In the case of Mill's system, pleasures and pains are divorced from their recipients and considered independently as contributing or not to the maximum happiness. The same point applies to Singer's interests since they are similarly divorced from their owners.

The second argument that is often used by consequentialists to counter the sort of criticism that we have put forward is that there is a disutility in allowing a situation where there is an unfair distribution in terms of benefits. In other words, more utility will be produced if there is a fairer distribution among individuals. However accurate this claim might be, the point still remains that individuals are not considered equally under a consequentialist interpretation. What is ultimately of value is the maximum production of what is considered to be good. If this in some cases allows for an unfair distribution then the consequentialists will have no way of condemning this. If enough benefit can be achieved, then it is possible that this might involve enormous harms to a small number of people since these harms will be outweighed by the total benefit.

Veatch constructed a hypothetical case where the greatest benefit would be achieved if 1% of the population were excluded from health care where this 1% comprises the:

> '... chronically ill with incurable illness, possessing insufficient intelligence to follow a medical regimen, and receiving expensive medical care'.[6]

The essence of the problem, then, for all these consequentialist theories is that they lose information about who is benefited and who is harmed and can only reflect the total benefits of a situation. As Veatch is highlighting, if those most in need were excluded from health care, the total amount of benefits would be increased. This point will be returned to later in the chapter when deontological interpretations of the Principle of Justice are considered.

6.2.3 QALYs and the allocation of medical resources

Before considering deontological interpretations of the Principle of Justice, we will illustrate the effects of a consequentialist approach to justice in the area of the allocation of health care resources (see 14.2).

Allocation of health care resources is undertaken at both the macro and micro level. The *macroallocation* level is where decisions are taken about how revenue should be distributed between the competing claims of, for example, health, education, defence, transport and arts. Decisions at this level are also taken when considering how to allocate resources within the health budget. For example, how much should be spent on mental health, community health, different treatments and different hospitals? The *microallocation* level is where one is determining which individuals should receive a certain treatment, for example, when there are only a limited amount of treatments available. What would count as a just distribution of the available treatments? The 'artificial hip example' is at this level.

A consequentialist approach to both the macro- and microallocation problems has been assumed by those who advocate adopting a quality adjusted life year (QALY) approach as a way of determining a just distribution of available resources.[7] Alan Williams stated that:

> '... the objective of economic appraisal is to ensure that as much benefit as possible is obtained from resources devoted to health care. In principle, the benefit is measured in terms of effect on life expectancy adjusted for quality of life'.[8]

Now, it is relatively uncontentious to say that we want as much benefit as possible from the resources allocated to health care. What is at issue is how we are to measure benefit. Williams proposes that benefit be measured in terms of how many QALYs can be obtained for the resources available. In other words, just as Mill argues that the best outcome is the greatest amount of happiness, Williams advocates that the best outcome is achieved when the greatest amount of QALYs is produced. They are both adopting a consequentialist approach, although they differ on what they take to have ultimate value.

Williams states that:

> '... the essence of a QALY is that it takes a year of healthy life expectancy to be worth 1, but regards a year of unhealthy life expectancy as worth less than 1. Its precise value is lower, the worse the quality of life of the unhealthy person (which is what the "quality adjusted" bit is all about). If being dead is worth zero, it is, in principle, possible for a QALY to be negative, i.e. for the quality of someone's life to be judged worse than being dead.'[9]

The only dimensions of quality that Williams has built into the concept of a QALY are those of physical mobility and freedom from pain. These evaluations were based on the responses of 70 'healthy' respondents. These evaluations, coupled with information about life expectancy, have yielded a meaning for the concept of a QALY. In addition, then, to objections to consequentialist accounts of justice, this particular consequentialist theory is operating with a very impoverished view of quality. It is one that assumes that qualitative dimensions ascertained from one group of the population can be extended to become universally applicable.[10]

At the macroallocation level, treatments are assessed according to the number of QALYs that they would yield coupled with the cost of these QALYs, which clearly vary from treatment to treatment. For example, the following figures were given by Williams:

> 'Heart transplantation yielding 4.5 QALYs at a cost of £5000 per QALY, kidney replacement yielding 5 QALYs at a cost of £3000 per QALY, and hip replacement yielding 4 QALYs at a cost of £750 per QALY.'[11]

On this basis, QALYs would be maximised by a transfer of resources to hip replacement treatments away from heart or kidney transplantation.

Is this a just way to allocate resources? Decisions at the macroallocation level clearly affect decisions at the microallocation level, since the former decisions determine how much money will be allocated to different parts of the health service. In addition, if a QALY approach is adopted at the microallocation level as well, this will immediately act to the disadvantage of those who have less life expectancy. One such group will be those who are old, which has led to the accusation that QALYs are ageist[12]. It will also act to the disadvantage of those who have conditions other than the one whose treatment is being contemplated. This is because they will register a lower score in terms of the QALY calculation. For example, an individual who needs a hip replacement and whose physical mobility is impaired by arthritis would score lower than the individual who just needs the hip replacement but does not have arthritis.

Although Williams has explored the concept of a QALY in more detail in later papers[13, 14], the above problems still apply. This is because they all illustrate the difficulties of allocating health care resources on the basis of QALY maximisation. The essence of the problem with any consequentialist account of what counts as a just distribution of available resources is that it does not take into account the needs of individuals. The primary reason for this is that the central concern for consequentialists is that outcomes be as good as possible and what counts as a good outcome is something that is divorced from the individual in the population who is receiving it. According to Mill we are seeking to maximise the quantity of happiness, for Singer the quantity of interest satisfaction, and for Williams the number of QALYs. These outcomes are judged in isolation from the question of which individuals receive these benefits.

Also, an implication of the particular consequentialist view adopted by Williams is that more QALYs will be yielded if treatments are given to those in less need since a larger amount of QALYs will be generated by this procedure. For example, someone who will die without a heart transplant needs that treatment more than someone who will not die without a hip replacement. However, as we have seen from the figures just given, QALYs will be maximised by hip replacements rather than heart transplants. What is needed is an account of justice that reflects the needs of individuals and does not act to the disadvantage of those who are in greatest need. We shall now look at a deontological approach to justice which does just this.

6.3 DEONTOLOGICAL INTERPRETATIONS OF JUSTICE

Rawls, in *A Theory of Justice*[15],proposes that we should determine what our principles of justice will be by imagining what principles we would choose from 'behind a veil of ignorance'. This 'veil of ignorance' reflects our ignorance of what position we will eventually hold within society. Since we do not know what natural attributes we will possess and in what social circumstances we will be placed, he considers that this device will produce a concept of justice as fairness. It is fair because it does not allow benefit to be distributed on the basis of accidental circumstances, for example, who one happens to be and into what social class one happens to have been born. He considers that this will lead to the position that we should distribute all vital economic goods and services equally, unless an unequal distribution would actually work to everyone's advantage. He arrives at two principles of justice which he initially formulates as:

> *First: each person is to have an equal right to the most extensive basic liberty compatible with a similar liberty for others. Second: social and economic inequalities are to be arranged so that they are both (a) reasonably expected to be to everyone's advantage, and (b) attached to positions and offices open to all.'* [16]

The principle of liberty given first is referring to those areas over which an individual ought to have autonomy. Areas that we have encountered in Chapter 4, such as freedom of thought, speech and combination with others. Political freedom and freedom to define life plans would also be included in this first principle. Rawls considers that this first principle has priority over the second. This is because the preservation of these liberties is not to be sacrificed to the goal of greater social or economic advantage. Liberty has intrinsic worth and is not being justified in terms of its recognition leading to a good outcome. This is the point of contrast between this deontological theory and consequentialist theories which only value liberty for the end that recognition of liberty might bring about (see 4.2.1). Rawls' deontological theory is taking the notion of what is right to be primary and not to be defined in terms of what will lead to good outcomes (see 2.3). This aspect of his theory leads him to give priority to the first principle since any social or economic gain cannot be justified at the expense of the denial of this first principle.

The two aspects of the second principle are also ordered such that '(b)' has priority over '(a)'. In other words, just as the second principle does not come into play until the first principle is satisfied, similarly, '(a)' is not applicable until '(b)' has been fully satisfied. As Rawls make clear later in his book, '(a)' is to guarantee that social and economic inequalities are arranged so that they are to the greatest benefit of the least advantaged (see also 17.7).

6.3.1 Illustration of Rawls' approach in health care

If we take an example at the macroallocation level the contrast between Rawls' approach and that incorporated in the consequentialist doctrine of QALYs is clearly illustrated. Let us suppose that there is a proposal to spend more money on the mentally retarded by withdrawing them from large, state-run institutions and instead housing them in smaller community based homes. Is it just to spend extra money on this section of the population? To simplify the case, we can assume that this extra money will be allocated from funds already made available to health spending. Therefore, there is no question of this claim on the money competing with expenditure claims in areas other than health.

It is claimed that the quality of life of the mentally retarded will be greatly improved if housed in these smaller units since the conditions in the large, state-run institutions are very poor. Ought the money to be spent on this programme? Alternatively, the money could be spent on health care for three other groups in society: normal or nearly normal children, adults of working age, and pregnant women. Many more normal or nearly normal children could be treated than in the former programme. Also, one product of health care for pregnant women would be less future children suffering from complaints such as Down's syndrome.

The object of considering this example is not to arrive at a decision to this particular case since many more details would have to be provided before that could sensibly be attempted. Rather, it is to illustrate the different *questions* that consequentialists would consider relevant to deciding this issue as opposed to adherents of deontological views. A consequentialist approach, such as that incorporated in the concept of a QALY, would consider the following questions to be relevant: How many QALYs would be yielded by each programme? What is the relative cost per QALY? It is likely that this sort of cost analysis would yield the result that the second programme should be adopted. However, adoption of the sort of deontological approach advocated by Rawls would make the following considerations relevant. It is important that those at present in the mental institutions have as much liberty as possible. Second, that as they are part of the least advantaged section of society, it should be recognised that any social and economic inequalities should be arranged to their greatest benefit. The needs of these individuals are being considered rather than concentrating on the greatest benefit that can be achieved irrespective of who receives that benefit.

6.4 CONCLUSION

What has emerged from these last three chapters on the Principles of Autonomy, Beneficence, Non-maleficence and Justice is the importance of valuing individuals in ethical decisions. Consequentialist justifications of all four of these principles take as central the value of outcomes. The maximisation of happiness, interest satisfaction, or QALYs is taken to be what is of value and the lives of individuals are only of secondary importance. Deontological justifications, on the other hand, value individuals as ends in their own right and not as means which can be traded off against one another as a means towards maximising some further end.

LEARNING EXERCISES

1. Ought equal consideration be given to individuals or to interests?
2. 'There are only limited resources to spend on health care. QALY calculations provide the fairest way of distributing these resources.' Do you agree or is it fairer to adopt Rawls' approach to the allocation of health care resources?

REFERENCES

1. Aristotle, *Nicomachean Ethics*, Book Five. In J.A.K Thomson (trans.) (1966) *The Ethics of Aristotle*. Penguin, London.
2. Mill, J.S. 'Utilitarianism'. In M. Warnock (ed.) *Utilitarianism*. Fontana Library, Glasgow, p319.
3. *Ibid*, p319.
4. Singer, P. (1933) *Practical Ethics* (2nd edn). Cambridge University Press, Cambridge, p21.
5. *Ibid*, p24.
6. Veatch, R. (1981) *A Theory of Medical Ethics*. Basic Books, New York, p172.
7. Goodinson, S.M. and Singleton, J. (1989) 'Quality of life: a critical review of current concepts, measures and their clinical implications'. *International Journal of Nursing Studies,* **26**: 4, 327–41.
8. Williams, A. (1985) 'Quality adjusted life years and coronary artery bypass grafting'. *DHSS Publication on Quality Adjusted Life Years 75–88*, p76.
9. *Ibid*, p78.
10. Goodinson and Singleton, *op. cit.*
11. Williams, *op. cit.*, p86.
12. Harris, J. 'More and Better Justice'.In J.M. Bell and S. Mendus (eds) (1988) *Philosophy and Medical Welfare*. Cambridge University Press, Cambridge.
13. Williams, A. 'Ethics and Efficiency in the Provision of Health Care'. In J.M. Bell and S. Mendus (eds) (1988) *Philosophy and Medical Welfare*. Cambridge University Press, Cambridge.
14. Williams, A. (1992) 'Cost-effectiveness analysis: is it ethical?' *Journal of Medical Ethics,* **18**: 7–11.
15. Rawls, J. (1976) *A Theory of Justice*. Oxford University Press, Oxford.
16. *Ibid*, p60.
17. Veatch, *op. cit.*, p252–3.

Key points

- The Principle of Justice. Equals ought to be considered equally.
- Mill's Principle of Justice. Equal amounts of happiness are equally desirable.
- Singer's Principle of Justice. Equal interests should be given equal consideration.
- The Principle of Declining Marginal Utility. 'For a given individual, a set amount of something is more useful when that individual has little of it than when he has a lot.'[5]
- Allocation of health care resources at the macroallocation level. How much revenue should be allocated to health care as opposed to education, defence, transport, etc. Also, within the health-care budget, how much money should be allocated to different treatments, hospitals, areas of health care, etc.?
- Allocation of health-care resources at the microallocation level. Which individuals should receive the available resources of the health-care system.
- A QALY. A year of healthy life expectancy is worth 1 and a year of unhealthy life expectancy is worth less than 1. The value is lower depending on the quality of life of the unhealthy person. At the macroallocation level, treatments are assessed in terms of their QALY yield and the cost per QALY. At the microallocation level, choices are made between individuals depending on how many QALYs are yielded by giving the treatment to a particular individual and the cost per QALY.
- Rawls' Principle of Justice[15]:
  1 'Each person is to have an equal right to the most extensive basic liberty compatible with a similar liberty for others.'
- 2. 'Social and economic inequalities are to be arranged so that they are both (a) reasonably expected to be to everyone's advantage, and (b) attached to positions and offices open to all.'

Acts and omissions, the Doctrine of Double Effect, and ordinary and extraordinary means

'To do nothing is in every man's power.'

Samuel Johnson (1709–84)

Learning outcomes

After reading this chapter, you should be able to:
- Understand how the acts and omissions doctrine would be treated within a consequentialist framework and a deontological framework.
- Evaluate whether there is a moral difference between acts and omissions.
- Understand and evaluate the Doctrine of Double Effect.
- Evaluate whether a distinction between ordinary and extraordinary means can yield morally significant conclusions.

7.1 ACTS AND OMISSIONS DOCTRINE

If we do not give as much to charity as we possibly could, we are allowing people to die. Is there any moral difference between this and killing someone? In general terms, is there any moral difference between acts and omissions?

7.1.1 Consequentialist view

In our discussion of the Principles of Beneficence and Non-maleficence we saw that consequentialists argue that there is no moral difference between actions and omissions (see 5.2.1). If we evaluate the rightness or wrongness of actions by their consequences then we must recognise that consequences can be produced by omissions as well as acts. This is why consequentialists support the view that there is a continuum between the Principles of Beneficence and Non-maleficence. Doing something to promote a benefit is at one end and omitting to harm is at the other. In both cases, it is the consequences that are important whether or not they are produced by an action or an omission.

One major problem with the denial of a moral difference between acts and omissions is that this would appear to make us just as responsible for those outcomes that result from what we do as those that result from what we omit to do. In not giving to charity, we are just as responsible for the death of those people that we allow to die as we would be if we went out and killed someone. As Glover writes:

> *'There is so much misery in the world that, however hard one person tries, he cannot remove more than a fraction. Does rejection of the acts and omissions doctrine commit us to being responsible for all that is left?'* [1]

Singer is quite prepared to accept this implication of consequentialism and argues in the specific case of death that there is no intrinsic moral difference between killing and allowing to die. In order to show that there is no *intrinsic* moral difference he considers two cases that are identical in all respects except that the first involves an omission and the second an action. The case study is adapted from one discussed by Sir Gustav Nossal, an eminent Australian medical researcher. The two cases can be summarised as follows.

The senile dementia example

An old lady of 83 has lost the ability to speak, requires to be fed, is incontinent, cannot sit up and is confined permanently to bed. She contracts pneumonia. She lives in a nursing home and her relatives are informed by the matron of the arrangements made for this type of case. With advanced senile dementia, they treat the first three infections with antibiotics, and after that, mindful of the adage that 'pneumonia is the old person's friend', they let nature take its course. The matron emphasises that if the relatives desire, all infections can be vigorously treated. The relatives agree to the former strategy. The patient dies of a urinary tract infection six months later.

The second case is identical to this, except that the patient is given a lethal injection. There is no difference in the amount of suffering of the patient. [2]

It must be remembered here that we are not constrained in our discussion by what is or is not allowed by the law at a particular time. Therefore it is inappropriate to raise the question of whether or not one would be liable to prosecution under present laws (see 1.5). Singer argues that since the outcomes in both these cases will be the same, there is no moral difference between them. The fact that one involved an omission and the other an action is not morally relevant. Of course, in many cases the outcomes will not be the same. Death as the result of omitting antibiotics is not likely to be so rapid as death as a result of a lethal injection. However, the assumptions of this example are that all features, other than one being an action and the other an omission, are the same.

Does this example show that there is no moral difference between actions and omissions in general and specifically that there is no difference in this particular case between killing and allowing to die? In this specific case we would agree with Singer that there is no moral difference between the two. However, to see if this point can be generalised to all cases of actions and omissions, it is necessary to examine the particular sort of omission that is in question in this example.

In the example described by Singer, the old lady's condition has been evaluated and a decision has been taken that the best outcome would be the death of the individual. In the first situation this outcome is achieved by not administering antibiotics in the event of an infection and in the second situation a lethal injection is used to achieve the outcome. The omission in this case, then, is the result of a conscious deliberation about the case, and might therefore more accurately be called an *act of omission*. The doctor in both cases is just as responsible for the death of the individual even though in the former case she omits to give antibiotics and in the latter she acts to give a lethal injection.

However, Singer is wrong to argue[3] that this then shows that in all cases there is no moral difference between killing and allowing to die. What we need to recognise is that there are different types of omission and that the act of omission, which is the result of a conscious deliberation, is not the only sort of omission. For example, there are those omissions that, far from resulting from deliberation, are the products of forgetfulness. In this sense, we might omit to switch off the lights on my car, which is not the result of a conscious decision but rather because I forgot that they were on. In these cases *the omission is unintentional*.

There are also omissions that do not fall into either of the above two classes, but comprise all those actions that could be said to have omitted because they are incompatible with the action actually performed. To take a trivial example, because I am typing at this moment I am omitting to do all actions other than typing, such as making a telephone call, going for a walk or gardening. This large class are all omissions in the sense *that I did not perform them*.

Consequentialists tend to assume that since they have shown that there is no moral difference between actions and omissions in cases where we have *intentional* acts of omission then it follows that there is never a moral difference between actions and omissions. In particular, they use this argument to support the claim that we should give more aid to those in the world who are dying. If we do not give more aid, that is, if we omit to give aid, then there is no moral difference between this and, for example, killing someone in the street. Irrespective of other arguments that might be advanced for why we should give more aid, this particular argument does not seem to work. For example, when we go out to buy a new colour television set we are not normally debating about whether to spend this money on a television set or on giving aid. Rather, this latter omission is the sort of omission that we described in the third case above. There are a large amount of acts that one omits to do simply because they are incompatible with the action that one is doing.

A famous quotation is often cited in support of there being a difference between killing and allowing to die. Clough writes:

> *Thou shalt have one God only; who*
> *Would be at the expense of two?*
> *No graven images may be*
> *Worshipped, except the currency*
>
> *'Thou shalt not kill, but need'st not strive*
> *Officiously to keep alive ...'* [4]

However, although these last two lines are often taken to be supporting a difference between acts and omissions, seen in the context of the whole poem, one can see that Clough's poem is satirical. Therefore he is really claiming that there is no difference between acts and omissions.

In fact, consequentialists would argue that in many actual cases, killing is preferable to allowing to die. These are cases where the effects of killing and allowing to die are not the same and, in these cases, killing may often be preferable to allowing to die. If it has been decided that the best outcome is the death of the individual, then it is often the case that there will be more pain and suffering for the individual, family and health carers if the individual is allowed to die rather than being killed. This is a valid point. Once a decision has been taken about what is best for an individual, then the option that involves the least pain and suffering is to be preferred. This conclusion is of course the reverse of what is generally accepted since allowing to die is thought to be preferable to killing.

7.1.2 DEONTOLOGICAL VIEW

The reason why deontologists support a difference between acts and omissions is because they hold that what makes an action right is the principle from which it has been done (see 2.3). This will explain why they could agree that there is no difference in the 'senile dementia example'. Here the principle guiding the action or omission is the same and therefore there is no moral difference between the two cases. However, in the case of omissions that I described as either being *unintentional* or falling under the class of actions *that I did not perform,* then the principle is not the same. I did not intend to leave my lights switched on and the principle governing my action of buying the television set was that I wanted to have the enjoyment of watching certain programmes.

Deontologists therefore will support the sort of criticisms that I have been making against consequentialist theories. Kant distinguishes between perfect duties, such as the duty of non-maleficence, and imperfect duties, such as the duty of beneficence (see 5.2.2). He argues that although the former allow of no exceptions, the latter are less stringent in the sense that it is up to us to decide whom we shall benefit. We are not in a position to benefit everyone unlike the duty of non-maleficence which is a duty that we owe universally. Consequently, it is inappropriate to blame individuals for omissions that fall into the third class of cases since it is up to them to decide whom they wish to benefit. Of course, we will encounter problems in some cases where the description of the case has been altered and the resulting description would determine whether or not it could be described as a duty of non-maleficence or beneficence (see 5.3).

7.2 THE DOCTRINE OF DOUBLE EFFECT

The point about how a situation can be variously described is at the centre of a criticism of the Doctrine of Double Effect. This doctrine states *that there is a difference between what one aims at (one's direct intention) and what is foreseen but is not intended (one's oblique intention).* Having drawn the distinction between intended consequences and foreseen consequences the claim is *that it is always wrong to do an action whose intended consequences are bad for the sake of foreseen consequences that are good, but that it may be permissible to perform an action whose intended consequences are good even though the foreseen consequences are bad.*

An example of this doctrine in use has been given by Foot. She writes:

> 'The operation of hysterectomy involves the death of the fetus as the foreseen but not strictly or directly intended consequence of the surgeon's act ... in another case, where a woman in labour will die unless a craniotomy operation is performed, the intervention is not to be condoned ... We foresee her death but do not directly intend it, whereas to crush the skull of the child would count as direct intention of its death.'[5]

Although this situation would not now normally occur since a delivery by Caesarean section is an option, this example highlights clearly the Doctrine of Double Effect.

According to the doctrine, the first case would be permissible. The second would not since the intended consequences, the crushing of the child's skull, would be bad and it is always wrong to perform an action whose intended consequences are bad for the sake of foreseen consequences that are good.

However, we need to ask what enables one to describe certain consequences as the intended consequences and others as the foreseen consequences of an action. This distinction appears to be dependent upon how the action is described in the first place. In the second example, if we described the action as one of saving the mother's life then the intended consequences would be that her life is saved and it is only a foreseen consequence that the fetus is killed. According to the Doctrine of Double Effect, this action would then become permissible. However, if it is described as an action whose intended consequences are the death of the fetus and it is only a foreseen consequence that the mother's life will be saved, then this action becomes wrong.

As we have seen earlier in other contexts, actions do not have unique descriptions. Unless there are restrictions on the legitimacy of certain descriptions of actions, the Doctrine of Double Effect will not be viable. However, if this is the case, it is surely wrong to argue that there is a moral difference dependent on whether an effect is foreseen or intended, when this latter distinction is dependent on a contingent decision about how to describe an action.

7.2.1 Implications for consequentialist theories

Rejection of the Doctrine of Double Effect means that Consequentialism will lead to some deeply counter intuitive results. As we noted earlier (see 5.2.2), the donation of the organs of one individual could save the lives of two people. If this was the case then consequentialists might have to argue that donation was the right action to perform since the consequences would be two individuals who are alive rather than one.

7.2.2 Implications for deontological theories

The Doctrine of Double Effect has been developed within the Roman Catholic tradition. It has been used to temper a deontological constraint, such as the prohibition against killing. For example, the termination of a pregnancy for a woman with a cancerous uterus is justified because the intended effect is to save the mother's life. The death of the fetus is only a foreseen consequence. Thus, this case is not described as a case of abortion.

It might be argued that there is an important distinction between the craniotomy example and the case of the cancerous uterus. In the former case, the crushing of the fetus' skull and thus the death of the fetus was necessary as a means towards achieving the end of saving the mother's life. However, in the case of the cancerous uterus, the death of the fetus is not essential as a means towards saving the mother's life. The removal of the fetus is essential but not the death of the fetus.

Therefore, in the craniotomy example part of the *intention* of the agent was that the baby's skull be crushed since this was needed as a means to the intended end. In this case, it could be argued, the baby's death is intended and not just foreseen. However, in the cancerous uterus example, although the removal of the fetus was part of the *intention* of the agent, the death of the fetus, if it occurred, was only foreseen and not intended.

This, though, will not save the doctrine. The death of the fetus in the craniotomy example may not be wanted or intended and regret for the death will be felt whether the cancerous uterus is removed or a craniotomy performed. In many cases, the results of both operations will be the death of the fetus, which highlights the artificiality of the distinction. If the act had been described as killing the fetus with the foreseen consequence that the mother's life would be saved, then this would not be allowable under the Doctrine of Double Effect.

7.3 ORDINARY AND EXTRAORDINARY MEANS

The distinction between ordinary and extraordinary means is often invoked as a way of determining whether or not it is legitimate to omit a particular treatment. It is considered that extraordinary treatments are morally optional whereas ordinary treatments are mandatory. In examining this claim we need to look first at what is meant by ordinary and extraordinary means. Second, we must consider whether or not the distinction provides a way of determining when a treatment is morally optional and when it is obligatory.

The discussion of ordinary and extraordinary means occurs frequently in discussions of euthanasia. It might be felt, for example, that while one should take all ordinary means to preserve life, one need not resort to extraordinary means. What does this mean? It might be assumed that by extraordinary means we are referring to complex medical apparatus that allows a life to continue. If this is the only way that the life can be sustained then it is not morally obligatory to keep the machine switched on since the life is only being preserved by extraordinary means. The assumption, then, is that by extraordinary means we mean sophisticated medical apparatus that is expensive and comparatively rare. In contrast, ordinary means refer to common and inexpensive treatments. If this is the case, does this distinction enable us to decide when a treatment is morally obligatory and when it is optional?

The answer would appear to be no. For example, if we take the giving of antibiotics this would fall into the class of ordinary means as defined above. Of course, it has not always been an ordinary means so it is evident that treatments that were once extraordinary might now be regarded as ordinary. What evaluation ought we to make about the case of an individual who is conscious and suffering from a painful and incurable disease and who then develops pneumonia? Ought this individual to be treated with antibiotics to cure the pneumonia? According to the definition of ordinary and extraordinary means just given, our answer to this question would be yes. Antibiotics are to be classed as ordinary means and therefore the treatment is obligatory. However, this does not seem to be the sort of consideration that is appropriate here. The question that needs to be considered is whether or not it is desirable that this individual's life be prolonged any further. This question needs to be answered *before* the question of means is considered. A definition that classifies treatments as ordinary or extraordinary cannot be used to *determine* answers to moral questions.

In fact, what this example makes clear is that the distinction between ordinary and extraordinary treatments cannot be said to classify different sorts of treatment. Rather, the different types of treatment are characterised as ordinary or extraordinary depending on the pain, benefit and expense in each individual case. What would count as an ordinary treatment in one case could be an extraordinary one in another case. In the example that we have just considered, it might well be decided that to administer antibiotics would be an extraordinary means given the evaluation of this individual's life. The distinction is therefore dependent on the evaluation of each case. It cannot be drawn prior to these evaluations and then used as a way of determining whether or not a treatment is morally obligatory or optional.

7.4 EVALUATION OF THE THREE DISTINCTIONS

Our ordinary moral thought reflects a distinction between acts and omissions which consequentialists are anxious to deny. The only thing of value for consequentialists is that outcomes be as good as possible. It is irrelevant, except where this makes a difference to the outcome, whether the consequences are produced by an action or an omission. We argue that this is correct in the case of omissions that are the result of conscious deliberation, but that there is a moral difference between actions and other sorts of omissions. Kant is right to argue that the duty of non-maleficence is a perfect duty whilst the duty of beneficence is an imperfect duty. We do not have a duty to benefit everyone and we are not responsible if we omit to do this. However, we do have a duty not to inflict harm on anyone, whether by a conscious deliberate action or by an omission.

The Doctrine of Double Effect has to be rejected since it is entirely dependent on how one decides to describe a particular action. Its rejection causes problems for consequentialism, since without it consequentialism could generate the judgement that great harms could be inflicted on individuals provided that the benefit to other individuals outweighed this harm.

Finally, a definition that enables us to classify treatments as either ordinary or extraordinary cannot be used to solve moral questions. The solution to moral questions comes first and the classification of treatments as either ordinary or extraordinary is dependent on, rather than the determinant of, moral evaluations.

LEARNING EXERCISES

1. The rightness or wrongness of an action is determined by the consequences of the action and it is morally irrelevant whether or not these consequences were produced by an act or omission. Critically discuss this view.

2. A woman proposes to have an abortion so that the fetal tissue can be used to save the life of a dying relative. Is this morally justifiable on the basis that her intention is to save the life of a dying relative and the death of the fetus is just a foreseen consequence?

REFERENCES

1. Glover, J. (1977) *Causing Death and Saving Lives*. Penguin Books, London, p104.
2. Singer, P. (1993) *Practical Ethics* (2nd edn). Cambridge University Press, Cambridge, pp207–8.
3. *Ibid*, p209.
4. Clough, A.H. (1977) *The Latest Decalogue*. Cited in Glover, *op. cit.*, p92.
5. Foot, P. 'The Problem of Abortion and the Doctrine of Double Effect'. In P. Foot (ed) (1978) *Virtues and Vices*. Blackwell, Oxford, pp20–1.

Key points

- By omitting to do as much as we can for others, we are allowing people to die. Is there any moral difference between this and killing people?
- The consequentialist view is that the rightness of actions is determined by their consequences. It is morally irrelevant whether these consequences were produced by actions or omissions.
- The Doctrine of Double Effect. There is a difference between what one aims at and what is foreseen but is not intended.
- Extraordinary treatments are optional and ordinary treatments are mandatory. Is this correct?

CHAPTER 8

A critical ethical approach to the problem of euthanasia

'It makes a great difference whether a man is lengthening his life or his death. If the body is useless for service, why should one not free the struggling soul?'

Seneca (?4 BC–AD 65)

Learning outcomes

After reading this chapter, you should be able to:
- Analyse a health-care dilemma using the discussion of the Principles in the previous chapters to assist you.
- Apply the four stages of analysis to specific principles that might be proposed. These are, isolation of principles, examination of the meaning of the principles, consideration of the implications of the principles and consideration of any change or qualification to the original principle.

8.1 THE PERSISTENT VEGETATIVE STATE (PVS) EXAMPLE

An individual, reliably diagnosed to be in PVS, has been in this state for several years. The close relatives of this individual and the attendant health care professionals consider that the best outcome for this individual is death. Should artificial nutrition and hydration be withdrawn from this individual in order that he might die?

The principles that have been discussed and the distinctions that have been drawn are now shown in use by considering the question of whether or not euthanasia is morally justifiable. The structure of the discussion is described in 3.3, and the relevance of the Principles of Beneficence, Non-maleficence, Autonomy and Justice are considered.

Euthanasia interpreted literally means a 'good death'. Current understanding of this term indicates that it is used to refer to a deliberate death brought about by one person for the benefit of another person, the person whose life is taken. There are at least two important points to note about this definition. First, euthanasia is distinguished from suicide since someone other than the person whose life is ended does the killing. Second, and more importantly, the death must be seen to be for the benefit of the person whose life is taken. This is crucial since some consequentialist justifications of euthanasia lead to cases where it might be deemed that the best consequences would be achieved if a person is killed, although there is no benefit to the person who dies. Thus we have Singer justifying euthanasia in cases where a 'disabled' infant could be replaced by another infant and thus bring about more happiness. He writes:

> 'When the death of a disabled infant will lead to the birth of another infant with better prospects of a happy life, the total amount of happiness will be greater if the disabled infant is killed.'[1]

This slide from genuine cases of euthanasia where the death is for the benefit of the person killed to cases which are justified on the grounds that the best consequences overall will be achieved by the death needs to be rejected. Taken to its extreme, it could lead to a utilitarian improvement policy where relatively minor 'defects' could be used as grounds for so-called 'euthanasia'. The assumption would be that a greater total benefit is achieved by the replacement of this infant by one not affected in the same way. This sort of argument is only used in cases of non-voluntary euthanasia, which is discussed later in the chapter.

As we mentioned in Chapter 1, our concern is whether cases of euthanasia can be morally justified. We are considering what ought to be the case and this might or might not be coincident with what is at present allowed by particular laws. Conversely, the moral rightness or wrongness of some action does not imply that this should be reflected in laws.

8.2 GLOVER'S GENERAL THEORY

To illustrate a critical ethical approach to this problem, we shall consider Glover's discussion of this issue in *Causing Death and Saving Lives*[2]. There are two reasons for taking this discussion as our focus point. The first is that he is adopting a non-cognitivist approach (see 3.2) and the second is that his treatment combines deontological and consequentialist principles. His adoption of non-cognitivism is illustrated when he writes:

> 'There is always the possibility, and sometimes the reality, of ultimate disagreement.'[3]

Moral judgements are expressions of our ultimate attitudes and hence, although there is room for rational discussion of ethical issues, there is still the possibility that there will not be agreement over ethical issues.

8.2.1 Isolation of Glover's principles

The first step in our critical ethical analysis is to isolate the principles that Glover is adopting (see 3.3.1). Isolation of the principles, examination of their meaning, analysis of their implications and the possible qualification of the original principles marks the four stages in the critical ethical approach that was discussed in Chapter 3.

Glover adopts two principles, one deontological and one consequentialist, which are concerned with the direct objections to killing. Direct objections are those that relate solely to the person killed. There are also side-effects of killing, where these are taken to be the effects on individuals other than the person killed. Glover does not provide any principles to deal with these, although he does note that by calling them side-effects we should not assume that they are less important than direct objections to killing. He writes:

> 'The direct objections to killing, although very strong, are not being presented here as ones that cannot be overridden ... It has not been argued that side-effects must always have less weight than the direct objections to killing.' [4]

The two principles governing the direct wrongness of killing are given by Glover as:

> 'A. It is wrong to reduce the length of a worth-while life.
> B. Except in the most extreme circumstances, it is wrong to kill someone who wants to go on living, even if there is reason to think this desire not in his own interests.' [5]

What do Glover's principles mean?

Principle B is referred to by Glover as the *Autonomy Principle* and he views it as having intrinsic worth. It is the deontological element in his account since the desire to carry on living is being valued even if there is reason to think that the consequences of this desire are not the best possible. Unlike Mill, Glover is not justifying his Autonomy Principle on consequentialist grounds (see 4.2.1). It is not a complete principle of autonomy since it is only concerned with the case of someone expressing the wish to go on living. A complete autonomy principle would cover all the desires of the individual.

Glover makes it explicit that not all human beings can be said to possess autonomy. For questions of autonomy to arise it is necessary for three conditions to be met. He describes these conditions as *the existence condition, the developmental condition and the possession condition*. The first condition is that the individual must already exist so that we cannot be said to be overriding the autonomy of potential individuals. Second, the individual must be sufficiently developed to be capable of the relevant desires. For example, someone like Singer would argue that young infants are not capable of having the desire to continue living since, although they are sentient, they are not yet 'persons' and hence self-conscious and rational. Finally, the possession condition states that the individual must actually have the relevant desire in question.

Principle A, on the other hand, is a consequentialist principle since the wrongness of killing is being explained in terms of it leading to the shortening of a worthwhile life. Glover considers that worthwhile lives are intrinsically valuable although he is not suggesting that everyone will share the same views about what makes life worthwhile. This will clearly vary from individual to individual.

Whenever more than one principle is proposed, unless they are ordered in terms of priority, there will always be the possibility of them conflicting in particular cases. There is no conflict between the principles as stated in the general theory but they could come into conflict in their application. Therefore, there is an indeterminacy in Glover's account at this point, since he does not provide an ordering for his two principles. He does, of course, insert the clause, 'except in the most extreme circumstances' in Principle B, but he is not claiming that Principle B always has priority over Principle A.

There is a further indeterminacy in Glover's general theory since there is nothing included in it about when direct objections to killing should override side-effects and when the opposite should be the case. He also does not, as we have already noted, provide any general principles to guide us in the consideration of side-effects.

8.1.3 What are the implications of Glover's principles?

Having considered these general points from Glover's theory, we now examine some implications of these principles when they are applied to the problem of euthanasia.

THE PROBLEM OF EUTHANASIA

How far will this general theory about killing take us in considering the problem of euthanasia? When discussing euthanasia it is usual to divide cases of euthanasia into three types. First we have *voluntary euthanasia.* This occurs when the individual has requested to die. An illustration of this would be the 'euthanasia example' in Chapter 1. There are problems with determining which cases fall into this category since there are two difficulties with this definition. First, is it limited to requests that are made at the time that the situation arises? Alternatively, can requests made earlier for what should happen to an individual in certain situations be considered as making this a case of voluntary euthanasia? This point is particularly pressing with the advent of 'living wills' in the US.

Second, what is to count as a 'request to die'? Does this request have to be made more than once? To whom should the request be made? The verification of whether or not the request is indeed an accurate reflection of what this individual wants is difficult to determine. The request might be based on faulty information about the quality of life that the individual can expect to enjoy if he or she does not end his or her life. Also, the request might just be a passing one felt, for example, when the individual was particularly depressed. It has also been argued that were euthanasia to become legal, individuals might feel pressurised into making requests to die from fear that they are becoming a burden on their families and not because they genuinely want to end their lives.

Setting these problems aside, if we assume that we do have a genuine case of voluntary euthanasia then how far will Glover's principles take us in the consideration of these sorts of cases? Glover argues that when we have a case of voluntary euthanasia, then both his principles apply. Strictly speaking, he is not entitled to claim that his autonomy principle applies since, as formulated, that only applies to requests to continue living. However, allowing this extension to requests to die to be included in the autonomy principle we then have cases where both principles are applicable. Therefore, we are confronted with the indeterminacy that is present in Glover's general theory concerning the ranking of the two principles. If we also assume that side-effects are always present in these sorts of cases, then we have the further indeterminacy of no principles governing side-effects. Also, there is no general way of ranking side-effects and direct objections to killing.

Although there is this indeterminacy in Glover's general theory, it would surely be naive to expect a moral theory to operate like a mathematical formula, where all one had to do is to enter in the features of the situation and then read off the moral conclusion. The assistance that Glover's theory provides is that it gives us a way of thinking about the problem. It gives us a way of distinguishing the different issues that are relevant. Also, we can see the problem in the wider context of being another case of killing alongside abortion, suicide and other life-and-death issues. He proposes the same principles for all life-and-death issues, which will assist in a consistent view being held about all these different dilemmas.

The theory is surely correct in the importance that it assigns to the Principle of Autonomy. First, it is given intrinsic worth and not justified on consequentialist grounds. Second, it claims that the Principle of Autonomy should only be overridden in 'the most extreme circumstances'. If we can be confident that the request for euthanasia is a genuine one, then the wish to die ought surely to be respected.

The second type of euthanasia is easier to deal with than voluntary euthanasia. This is *involuntary euthanasia* and is defined as euthanasia where the individual in question has not expressed the wish to die. For this to be classed as a case of euthanasia and not murder it must be understood that although the individual has not expressed a wish to die, it is thought to be in that individual's best interests that he or she should die. Appeal is therefore being made to a Principle of Beneficence coupled with a paternalistic evaluation of what is of benefit to the individual (see 5.5).These are cases where we have individuals who are capable of making or not making requests to die and have either explicitly asked not to die or they have just not requested death. Clearly, if any justification for involuntary euthanasia is possible, it will be based on consequentialist grounds. It is assumed that the consequences of continuing living will not be a worthwhile life. Both Glover's principles apply, but the autonomy principle is overridden since it is assumed that someone else, other than the individual concerned, can better evaluate what makes that individual's life worth living. It is extremely unlikely that this paternalistic class of cases of euthanasia could ever be justified and the only conceivable case that Glover constructs is not likely to provide a sufficient justification given the uncertainty governing future events[6].

Arguably, the most difficult cases of euthanasia are those that fall into the class of *non-voluntary euthanasia.* The 'persistent vegetative state' example with which we started this chapter is an illustration of this. These are cases where the individual has no views about the continuation of their life, either because they are, for example, babies or because they are not in a position to communicate such views, for example, if they are in a coma. In these cases the only principle that is relevant is the Worthwhile Life Principle, since the Principle of Autonomy will not be applicable. Although the existence condition for autonomy will be met, the individual does not possess or is not capable of communicating the desire to either continue or not continue living. In Singer's sense of the term, the individual is not a 'person'.

In one sense, the lack of applicability of the Principle of Autonomy might appear to make these cases easier, since there is no possibility of conflict between the two principles. There is, of course, still the consideration of side-effects to be taken into account and these might conflict with the Worthwhile Life Principle, but one potential source of conflict has been removed. However, despite the removal of this potential area for conflict, these cases are still the most intractable of the three.

There are tremendous difficulties in determining whether or not an individual's life is worth living. In addition to the uncertainty of how accurate their future prospects are taken to be, there is the whole question of how these should be evaluated with reference to this particular individual. Also, who ought to make this evaluation? Should it be a member of the health care team or a close relative of the individual? The health care team are probably in a better position to predict the physical conditions that an individual will be placed in, but it is more likely that a close relative of the individual would be in a better position to evaluate what these conditions would mean to the individual in question. Expertise in health care does not automatically provide one with expertise to make these evaluations.

Even if we assume that we have a case where we are as certain as we can be that the individual's life is not worthwhile, it is still an open question whether that individual ought to be killed. For example, there are those that support a *Sanctity of Life Principle* who would argue that even if it is accepted that this individual's life is not worthwhile, life itself is of value and should not be destroyed. Now, in cases of non-voluntary euthanasia the most that we have are lives that are merely conscious and sometimes we do not even have this. The individual in the 'persistent vegetative example' was not even conscious. Since we have assumed in this class of cases that the life involved would not be a worthwhile life, adherents to the Sanctity of Life Principle can only be valuing, at most, mere consciousness. The question then arises, does mere consciousness have intrinsic value or is it only of value because of what it might lead to?

If you argue that mere consciousness as such has intrinsic value then you are arguing that dimensions such as sight, hearing and smell are of intrinsic value. They are of value in themselves and not because of what they might lead to. However, an implication of this sort of view that there are no grounds for giving priority to the life of a human being as opposed to that of many other species since they also possess these features of consciousness. This might not be an implication that some people find acceptable, since they consider that human life is of more value than the life of other species. However, someone like Singer would be quite prepared to accept this implication, since he claims that what is of importance is the possession of consciousness and not what species is involved (see 3.4).

Those who wish to continue claiming that the consciousness of human beings is of more value than that of other species might do so by arguing that consciousness in human beings has a greater potential for becoming more than mere consciousness. However, if this claim is made, it would contradict the previous claim than consciousness has intrinsic value. This is because the superiority of human consciousness is being supported on the grounds that it is instrumental to something else whereas the original claim was that consciousness had intrinsic value. Also, in the example we are considering, we assume that we do not have anything else, that we do not have a worthwhile life. Hence, if one holds that consciousness has intrinsic worth it would seem that one would have to accept that there are no grounds for giving priority to human beings as a species. Indeed, there might be certain cases where priority could be given to members of other species on the grounds that their level of consciousness is superior. A human being who lacked sight and hearing might, on these arguments, be accorded less value than a member of another species with the full complement of consciousness.

In the previous section we assumed that the individual's life was not worthwhile. However, surely one of the most important questions in cases of non-voluntary euthanasia is to determine how we are going to establish whether or not an individual's life is worthwhile. Glover suggests that the best procedure is to put yourself in the other individual's position and consider the question from his or her point of view. But how is this to be done? It is surely not possible to achieve a complete identification with all the preferences of another individual but, if this is not the case, what preferences of one's own does one retain? Also, there is one preference that the individual by definition does not have and that is the preference about whether or not they want their life to continue or not. In other words, the evaluation will still be your own and it is on this basis that you will determine whether or not the individual's life is worthwhile.

Let us now assume that we are confident that the life in question is not worthwhile and that we have rejected the sanctity of life principle. What ought we to do in these sorts of cases? A standard reply might be that given that the life is judged not to be worthwhile then all *ordinary means* ought to be taken to preserve life but that we need not resort to *extraordinary means*. However, we have argued (see 7.3) that the distinction between ordinary and extraordinary means is not a distinction that can be drawn between particular treatments. It is a distinction that can only be drawn after the value questions about someone's life have been settled. Of how much value is it that this life be continued since we have assumed that it is not worthwhile? We have to compare this with the side-effects of keeping this individual alive. Side-effects include the effects on the carers, relatives and other individuals requiring medical resources which might otherwise be used on this individual. It is in connection with this last point that the Principle of Justice becomes relevant to the discussion. In the context of scarce health care resources, how much money ought to be allocated to the prolongation of merely conscious or permanently unconscious lives? It is answers to these sort of questions that enable us to describe a particular procedure as being ordinary or extraordinary. The treatments themselves are only described as ordinary or extraordinary once the value questions described have been answered.

Another reply might be to say that given that this individual's life is not worthwhile, we will not take any active procedures to kill him but we will take no steps to preserve the individual's life. This reply is based on there being a distinction between *acts and omissions*. In this sort of case the omission would be the result of a conscious decision and it would be more appropriate to describe it as an act of omission. In the case of omissions of this sort, we argued in 7.1.1 that there was no intrinsic moral difference between these and acts. Therefore, given that we have agreed that this individual's life is not worthwhile, omitting treatments to preserve his or her life is the same as actively killing him if the consequences are the same. Of course, in many cases the consequences will not be the same and usually, in terms of lack of pain for the individual, there will be less pain as a result of active procedures than by omitting treatment.

A third reply in this sort of case might be to argue that we are justified in performing an action that has death as a *foreseen consequence* but not as an *intended consequence*. For example, we might advocate the use of very powerful pain killers with the intended effect of alleviating pain but whose foreseen consequences is the death of the individual. However, as we argued 7.2, the distinction between intended and foreseen consequences is dependent on a contingent decision about how one describes the situation. Moral evaluations cannot be made dependent on how one decides to describe a situation.

Presumably, if it is decided that the individual's life is not worthwhile and that death is the best outcome for that individual, then the only other considerations that are necessary to raise before killing the individual are the side-effects of this action. The side-effects include not only the effects on the relatives and health care team but also the effects on society at large if euthanasia were practised in these sort of cases. The consideration of side-effects might well lead one to adopt the policy of giving the pain killer which will ultimately lead to the death of the individual rather than performing a direct act of killing. However, this decision would not be based on a distinction between intended and foreseen consequences but would be the result of balancing the side-effects and direct objections to killing.

LEARNING EXERCISES

1. 'It is wrong to terminate life because life is sacred.' Critically assess this view by subjecting the principle of the sanctity of life to the four stages of discussion illustrated in this chapter. You might find it helpful to refer back to Chapter 3 where these stages were first discussed.

REFERENCES

1. Singer, P. (1993) *Practical Ethics* (2nd edn). Cambridge University Press, Cambridge, p186.
2. Glover, J. (1977) *Causing Death and Saving Lives*. Penguin Books, London.
3. *Ibid*, p35.
4. *Ibid*, p115.
5. *Ibid*, p113.
6. *Ibid*, pp191–2.

Key points
- Glover's two principles governing the direct wrongness of killing:
  A. It is wrong to reduce the length of a worthwhile life.
  B. Except in the most extreme circumstances, it is wrong to kill someone who wants to go on living, even if there is reason to think this desire not in his own interests.[5]
- Glover's three conditions for autonomy: existence, development and possession.
- Voluntary euthanasia. The individual has requested to die.
- Involuntary euthanasia. The individual has not expressed a wish to die.
- Non-voluntary euthanasia. The individual has no views on the continuation of their life either because they have never been in a position to have these views or because they did not express their views when they were capable of expressing them.
- Sanctity of Life Principle. Life is of value and should not be destroyed.
- If a life is judged not to be worthwhile, ought all *ordinary* means be taken to preserve that life, but not *extraordinary* means?
- The Principle of Justice. How much money is it fair to allocate to the prolongation of permanently unconscious lives?
- If an individual's life is not worthwhile, we take no active measures to kill him or her, but we will take no steps to preserve his or her life. Is this a viable position?
- If an individual's life is not worthwhile, we will not kill him or her intentionally, but have as our intention the relief of his or her pain by powerful pain killers, although the foreseen consequences will be his or her death. Is this a viable postion?

SECTION 2

CONTEMPORARY HEALTH CARE DILEMMAS

Definitions of life and death

Definition of life: 'The continuous adjustment of internal relations to external relations.'

H. Spenser (1820–1903)

Learning outcomes

After reading this chapter, you should be able to:
- Understand and evaluate the five views presented of life and death at the end of life.
- Understand and evaluate the conservative view of life at the beginning of life.
- Understand and evaluate the person view of life at the beginning of life.
- Understand and evaluate the potential human being view at the beginning of life.

9.1 THE PROBLEMS

We have shown how the distinctions that were introduced in Section 1 can be used to assist analysis of the problem of euthanasia. Clearly, a fundamental issue that is related not only to euthanasia but also to organ donation, decisions about resuscitation, abortion, contraception, the use of fetal tissue and many more related areas, is how to define life and death. We need an analysis of the concepts of life and death in order to clarify our views about these issues and to ensure that a consistent view of life and death is being held over the whole range of these issues. A definition that is considered acceptable from one perspective might have to be rejected when the implications of this definition are appreciated in other life-and-death issues.

Another question that has to be addressed is the question of the relationship between the concepts of life and death as they are used at the beginning and end of life. Is it the case that concepts developed for use at the end of life, for example, can also be used at the beginning of life? If they cannot, what are the relevant differences between the end of life and the beginning of life that make it inappropriate to use the same concepts in each case?

In these discussions we shall also have to bear in mind why we need definitions of life and death. Reasons have already been given and, in addition, there are social, psychological and legal reasons why these questions are important. Individuals need to know when, for example, a close relative is still alive or dead for legal reasons and also in terms of their relationship to this relative.

Finally, it should not be assumed that we are just looking for definitions of 'life' and 'death' which can then be used to assist in the solution of ethical problems. The definitions that are chosen presuppose solutions to value questions. The definitions themselves result from ethical decisions about how to answer questions of life and death. The definitions incorporate these evaluations and must not be regarded as evaluatively neutral.

For example, let us take the 'persistent vegetative state example' discussed in Chapter 8. If we call this individual 'dead' this will not remove a problem. Allocating the term 'dead' to the condition of permanent unconsciousness indicates an evaluation of this condition. It is the end result of an evaluation rather than a starting point to be used to settle value questions.

9.2 DEFINITIONS OF LIFE AND DEATH

When considering various proposed definitions of life and death it is important to understand the perspective from which they have been developed. We shall argue that definitions of death should be developed which are in the interests of the individual affected. In other words, it is inappropriate to define death, for example, in terms of what will produce the best outcome for organ donation or in terms of the financial cost of not allowing certain conditions to be described as death. Thus a consequentialist account of death which seeks a definition that leads to the best outcome being achieved for everyone affected in the situation will be rejected. Rather, a deontological concept of death is needed. Here the individual is being considered as, in Kant's terms (see 4.2.2), an end in him or herself and is not being considered as a means towards the best outcome being achieved (see 15.3.3).

There are two main questions to distinguish when looking at the concepts of both life and death. First, there is the conceptual issue of what is intended by the terms 'life' and 'death'. Second, there is the question of whether there are clear empirical criteria that can be used to reflect the conceptual analyses of life and death. For example, if it is argued that 'death' means permanent loss of consciousness, then it would be a separate question to consider how this state might be identified in an individual. These questions are not always clearly distinguished and, where they are, sometimes answers to the second question are used to reinforce a particular conceptual analysis.

9.2.1 Life and death at the end of life

There seem to be five major candidates for consideration in the conceptual analysis of life and death. We describe them by considering those theories first that demand the most in terms of what is to be counted as being alive and proceed to those that allow a very minimalist concept of life. The first group of theories, which we call the 'Person View', concentrate on what is of value in life and argue that what gives life value is the sum of one's aspirations, decisions, activities, projects and human relationships.[1]

Rachels, who holds this view, talks about the possession of these characteristics constituting what counts as being alive in a biographical sense as opposed to being alive in a biological sense. Although it is necessary to be alive in the biological sense in order to have a biographical life, the former is not sufficient for a biographical life. Many species of animals whilst alive in the biological sense are not capable of sustaining a biographical life. Being alive in the biographical sense seems largely to correspond to Singer's notion of being a person (see 3.4.2) and as such is not limited to human beings. Indeed, Rachels writes:

> 'When we consider the mammals with which we are most familiar, it is reasonable to believe that they do have lives in the biographical sense.'[2]

Rachels makes it clear that although consciousness is a necessary condition for a biographical life it is not sufficient. He describes a case, typical of many others[3], where an individual, who had suffered brain injury at birth, was practically mindless, blind, mute and deformed in all limbs. Although he was conscious and could feel pleasure and pain, he did not have a life in the biographical sense since:

> '... the sensations experienced will not be endowed with any significance by the one experiencing them; they will not arise from any human activities or projects; they will not be connected with any coherent view of the world.'[4]

Another condition that is also presented as being necessary for having a life in a biographical sense is memory. Rachels cites the example of an individual who has no memory of anything that happened after he was 19 in 1945. Rachels writes:

> 'Without the continuity that memory makes possible, a life, in any but the most rudimentary sense, is unattainable.'[5]

This is, of course, Rachel's evaluation of this case, which would not necessarily be coincident with the view taken by the individual in question. Rachel's view is in line with Singer's definition of a person since a necessary condition of being self-conscious is that one has some idea of a self continuing over time.

Therefore, individuals in a persistent vegetative state and individuals who are merely conscious and who do not have the extra characteristics necessary to make them capable of biographical lives will be alive biologically, but they will not possess those characteristics that make lives of value. In the famous case of Karen Quinlan, who was in a persistent vegetative state, Rachels writes:

> '... continued biological existence is almost certainly not a benefit'.[6]

Having elucidated these concepts of life and death one would expect that the criteria that Rachels would advance for death would be those that corresponded with the loss of biographical lives. However, Rachels puts forward a more modest proposal and argues that the time of death should be fixed at the point where consciousness is no longer possible and he claims that the criterion for this is brain death. This, as we shall see, is not entirely clear, but his proposal apparently leads one to classify those in a permanent vegetative state as being dead. Rachels writes:

> *'... this means that "brain death" precludes any restoration of consciousness: at that point, we can be sure the donor's organs are no longer of any use to him. So, it is morally all right to fix the time of death at that point.'* [7]

The second group of views are those that hold that life, at least for human beings, corresponds to the capacity for consciousness. This is what is important for human life and without it the individual can be said to be dead. This view that the identity of a person ceases with their loss of capacity for consciousness, at which point they can be regarded as dead, is held by, amongst others, Green and Wikler.[8]

The criterion proposed to reflect this state is loss of higher brain functioning. How this can be determined is still problematic, although positron emission tomographic (PET) scanning techniques have been used to try to determine this[9]. Again, this means that those individuals in a persistent vegetative state are regarded as dead and we would have the problem, as Gervais notes, of:

> *'How shall we manage patients who are demonstrably in persistent vegetative states, once we have declared them dead?'* [10]

As the law stands, disposal of the body in this state could not take place.

The third group of views are those that argue that whilst any of the minimum conditions for life remain, the individual is still alive. Lamb writes:

> *'The minimum requirements for human life are the capacity for consciousness and the capacity for respiration and heartbeat.'* [11]

He argues that cessation of these capacities counts as death since death is:

> *'... the irreversible loss of function of the organism as a whole'.* [12]

Bodily integration is what is constitutive of human life and loss of these capacities is equivalent to a lack of this integration.

This account of the concept of death yields, according to Lamb, clear empirical criteria for determining death:

> *'... irreversible loss of brainstem function necessarily involves loss of both the capacity for consciousness and the capacity to breathe'.* [13]

The upper brainstem is responsible for the capacity for consciousness and the lower brainstem is responsible for the capacity for respiration and heartbeat. He notes that it is important that brainstem dysfunction is contextually determined to remove the possibility of other causes for this which would not be irreversible. Causes such as hypothermia and drug intoxication have to be eliminated.[14]

One of the implications of this definition is that individuals who are in a persistent vegetative state, having lost most if not all of the higher brainstem function, will still be classified as being alive. Although the capacity for consciousness is lost, the individual is still deemed to be alive. This is arguably the central point of difference between this concept of death and the first two accounts. This point is obscured by

Rachels' use of the phrase 'brain death' as equivalent to the cessation of the capacity for consciousness.

The fourth view includes even more states in what could be regarded as being alive than the third view. This fourth view has recently been advocated by the Danish Council of Ethics and it is claimed that it is a concept of death that is in line with what individuals expect in their everyday experience of death. In this everyday experience, it is claimed that:

> '... the process of death cannot be said to have ended while respiration and heartbeat continue, the body remains warm and the colours of the body normal. Such a state is, of course, compatible with brain death, and few people would be prepared to refer to a body in this state as a "corpse".' [15]

This concept, which allegedly reflects the ordinary experience of death, thus generates cardiac-oriented criteria for death. Of all the proposals considered, this definition clearly gives the widest scope to what counts as life.

Lastly, a fifth group of views encompasses spiritual concepts related to the process of dying, and can be a reflection of individual beliefs. These could allow even more states to be included in the concept of 'life' than the fourth view. For example, in Tibetan Buddhism, the process of dying is considered to comprise two phases of dissolution. An outer dissolution occurs, during which the senses and physical functions deteriorate, culminating in the cessation of respiration and circulation. An internal process, 'inner respiration', continues for approximately 20 minutes. A phase of inner dissolution of thought and emotions also occurs, during which four increasingly subtle levels of consciousness are encountered.[16] Although variable, the view is held that it can take up to three days for consciousness to separate from the body.

Evaluation of these proposals

Having stated these five groups of views, it is clear how important it is to either decide between them or to propose an alternative. This decision will, for example, affect how we regard organ transplants, whether or not they are being taken from an individual who is alive or dead. Also whether or not it is appropriate to consider euthanasia will be determined by whether or not the individual is already deemed to be dead anyway.

It is clearly important to reach agreement on a concept of death before formulating empirical criteria that will reflect this concept. What it means to be alive and dead raises philosophical issues about the essence of lives. However, it is also important that one has a concept of death that can be reflected in clear empirical criteria. Lamb's proposal appears to satisfy this latter point as there are clear tests for establishing brainstem death.[17] On the other hand, loss of the capacity for consciousness does not yield clear unambiguous criteria.

However, although one might be prepared to accept Lamb's concept of death, the points made by the first and second view are clearly extremely important. Even if we are not prepared to count as dead those individuals in a persistent vegetative state or, similarly, anencephalic infants, the first two conceptions concentrate on issues that are important to the question of non-voluntary euthanasia (see 8.2.3). We need to consider what gives value to life to determine whether there is any sense in which these individuals have lives of value. It is not a case of pronouncing them dead by definition but it highlights the difference that needs to be drawn between just being alive and having a life of value. This is an evaluative question that needs to be considered and cannot be prejudged by proposing to include these states in what is to count as dead. Indeed, if we adopted this proposal, we would be presented with the problem of how to deal with those individuals who are in a persistent vegetative state and are on this view considered to be dead. Gervais suggests that we manage these individuals by:

> '... a simple act with an immediate result – for example, an injection of potassium chloride'.[18]

The fourth view advocated by the Danish Council of Ethics appears to allow too much to the concept of life. It recognises that brainstem death is irreversible and indeed marks the beginning of the death process but does not allow it to be constitutive of death. However, it does not seem conceivable that continued existence of the individual after brainstem death can be in the interests of that individual at all.

The fifth group of views highlights a possible objection to this last point. If the individual was known to have spiritual beliefs which include a view of death such as illustrated in the Buddhism example, then these views should be respected.

9.4 LIFE AND DEATH AT THE BEGINNING OF LIFE

When does life begin? In the above discussion we consider the cessation of life and when it is appropriate to describe someone as dead. Is the concept of life that we have accepted here acceptable as an account of when life can be said to have begun? It has been argued that the converse notion of brain birth is not a helpful way to determine the beginning of life.[19] (See 15.3.3)

One possible reason for why it is inappropriate to expect that the meaning of the term 'life' will be regarded in the same way at the beginning and end of lives is that the beginning of life marks the start of a process that has the *potential* for developing into what Rachels would describe as a 'biographical life'. On the other hand, the end of life is something that is *irreversible* and indicates the loss of features that can never be regained.

Another reason that might be considered is in terms of why we need an account of when life begins. An answer to this question is necessary when considering the justifiability or otherwise of issues such as abortion, embryonic research, use of fetal tissue and *in vitro* fertilisation. Some of these issues are different from those that arise at the end of life and might necessitate a different concept of life. This is not to say that we need a definition of life that will be justified in consequentialist terms. One that what will produce, for example, the greatest benefit in terms of embryonic research. Rather, the point is that the need for the clarification of the concept of life arises in a different context at the beginning of life than at the end of life.

The majority of views hold that life begins at fertilisation, but they differ in the status that they ascribe to the life that has begun. Therefore, the important question becomes, what status do we attribute to the embryo and subsequent fetus? The conservative view holds that the embryo must be regarded in the same way that we regard other members of our species that have been born. One argument that is advanced for this view is that the development of the embryo through the fetal stage to eventual birth is a continuous process which does not have any stages that can be regarded as morally significant from the point of view of the status of the being. Various points in this development have been suggested as being morally significant and as providing a justification of according the fetus a different status to adult human beings, but these can all be rejected according to the conservative view.

One point that has been taken to have moral significance has been birth. This is, of course, a point that is taken to be significant from a legal point of view. Neonates are accorded a different status from the developing fetus.[20] However, it has been pointed out that this would have the consequence of according a different status to the premature baby as opposed to the fetus at the same stage of development, but who had not been born. This seems clearly inconsistent and the conservative view is right to reject birth as being a morally significant dividing line.

Another point in the development of the fetus that has been suggested to be morally relevant is the point at which the fetus becomes viable, that is, able to live outside the uterus. However, again the conservative view is surely right when it rejects this argument. The grounds for rejection are that the date of viability has not only changed over the years but also varies depending on the location of the pregnant woman and what medical facilities are in close proximity. Contingent factors such as these should not determine the moral status of the fetus.

Quickening, when the mother first feels the fetus move, has also been proposed as a point where a different moral status could be accorded to the fetus. However, this is arguably the least likely candidate since this awareness is extremely variable from mother to mother.

Another point which has been taken to be significant is brain birth so that, just as at the end of life brain death constitutes death, so at the beginning of life brain birth provides a morally significant stage. However, as with other developments, brain birth is a gradual process, with different regions of the brain developing at different times, and there is therefore no simple point that can be indicated where brain birth occurs.[21]

A final suggestion that has come to prominence with the publication of the Warnock Report is that 14 days from fertilisation marks a morally significant dividing point in the development of the embryo. This is because at about 15 days we have the formation of the primitive streak and this is the latest stage at which two individuals (identical twins) could develop rather than one. The primitive streak is the first identifiable feature within the embryonic disc. It should be emphasised that the only reason for specifying an exact number of days rather than opting for a less specific demarcation of this stage was that legislation necessitated a clear unambiguous demarcation point.[22]

However, like all the other dividing lines that have been suggested, this does not seem to have moral significance, since essentially the process from fertilisation to birth is a continuous process. The fact that there might be more than one individual up to this point does not alter the moral status of the embryo but is indicative that this process of development might result in two individuals rather than one.

Therefore, the conservative view is right to argue that there are no morally significant dividing lines in the process from fertilisation to birth. However, whilst accepting this aspect of the conservative view, it does not follow that one is obliged to accept that the embryo and resulting fetus have the same status as an adult human being.

A view, which we might call the person view, denies that the fetus has the same status as that of an adult human being and is held by, amongst others, Singer (see 3.4). He suggests that we look at the actual state of the fetus in the context of his consequentialist moral principle that the right action to perform is that action which will maximise the interests of those affected in a situation. Since the embryo does not have interests as it lacks the capacity for sentience, the embryo and fetus up to a certain point of development will not have to figure in moral calculations. Although the fetus will never achieve the status of a 'person', it will during its development acquire the capacity for consciousness and at that point will possess interests that have to be taken into account. It is interesting to note that Singer writes that the:

> '... search for a morally crucial dividing line between the newborn baby and the fetus has failed ... The conservative is on solid ground in insisting that the development from the embryo to the infant is a gradual process.' [23]

However, Singer's view itself does involve drawing morally significant dividing lines, since he distinguishes between the sentient and non-sentient fetus.

There are other views that we will discuss specifically when we discuss abortion, but the final view about life to be discussed in this chapter is the view that the fetus from the moment of conception should be regarded as a potential human being. In order to consider fully which view is acceptable, the implications for this and the other views in all areas in which they are relevant have to be considered and this is what will be done in subsequent areas of the book when discussing such issues as abortion and embryonic research (see Chapter 3).

The first point to note about this view is that it clearly denies that we just look at the actual characteristics of the embryo or fetus. We consider the embryo or fetus as having the potential to develop into a fully grown member of our species. In Singer's terms, it is a member of a species that can have 'persons' as its members and it is therefore inappropriate to ignore this and just consider its actual characteristics.

It may be objected that if we accord this status to the embryo and fetus, then we shall have no way of limiting our starting point to conception since, it might be claimed, the sperm and ova similarly have the potential to become human beings. This might be regarded as an objection especially in the light of what it might entail for views about contraception (see 3.3.4). However, it can be countered that neither the sperm nor egg separately have the status of being potential human beings, since neither, by itself, could develop into a human being.

A decision regarding which, if any, of these views regarding life and death ought to be accepted should be deferred until the implications of these views is worked out, which is undertaken in the following chapters. We need a view about life and death that can be held consistently through the different range of issues that rely on these concepts.

LEARNING EXERCISES

1. How ought we to treat individuals who are in a permanent vegetative state?
2. Is there a morally significant dividing line in the development of the fetus from conception?

REFERENCES

1. Rachels, J. (1986) *The End Of Life*. Oxford University Press, Oxford, p26.
2. *Ibid*, p35.
3. *Ibid*, p29.
4. *Ibid*, p30.
5. *Ibid*, p53.
6. *Ibid*, p99.
7. *Ibid*, p43.
8. Green, M.B. and Wikler, D. 'Brain Death and Personal Identity'. In M. Cohen, T. Nagel and T. Scanlon (eds) *Medicine and Moral Philosophy*. Princeton University Press, New Jersey, pp49–77.
9. Levy, D., Sidtis, J., Rottenberg, A., Jarden, J., Strother, S., Dhawen, V., Tramo, M., Evans, A. and Plum, F. (1987) 'Differences in cerebral blood flow and glucose utilization in vegetative states as opposed to locked-in patients'. *Annals of Neurology*, **22**(6): 673–82.
10. Gervais, K. (1987) *Redefining Death*. Yale University Press, New Haven, p176.
11. Lamb, D. (1985) *Death, Brain Death and Ethics*. Croom Helm, London p7.
12. *Ibid*, p14.
13. *Ibid*, p36.
14. *Ibid*, p34.
15. Rix, B. (1990) 'Danish ethics council rejects brain death as the criterion of death'. *Journal of Medical Ethics*, **16**: 5–7.
16. Rinpoche, S. (1992) *The Tibetan Book of Living and Dying*. Rider Books, London.
17. Lamb, *op. cit.*, p53.
18. Gervais, K., *op. cit.*, p176.
19. Jones, D.G. (1989) 'Brain birth and personal identity. *Journal of Medical Ethics*, **15**:173–8.
20. BMA (199) 'A "neonate" is defined as "a newly born infant under the age of one month'. In *British Medical Association Reference Guide on Family Health*. Dorling Kindersley, London.
21. Jones, *op. cit.*
22. Warnock, M. (1985) *A Question of Life: The Warnock Report on Human Fertilisation and Embryology*. Basil Blackwell, Oxford, ppxv–xvi.
23. Singer, P. (1993) *Practical Ethics* (2nd edn). Cambridge University Press, Cambridge, pp142–3.

Key points
- Person View. Biographical lives are what is important, not biological lives. Biographical lives are those where one has the capacity to pursue activities, have projects and form relationships.
- Consciousness View. Life corresponds to the capacity for consciousness.
- Human life corresponds to the capacity for consciousness and the capacity for respiration and heartbeat.
- Danish Council of Ethics advocates that life corresponds to continued respiration and heartbeat.
- Spiritual Views. These may allow even more states to be included in what it is to be alive.
- Conservative View. The embryo must be regarded in the same way that we treat other members of our species.
- Is birth morally significant?
- Is the viability of the fetus morally significant?
- Is quickening morally significant?
- Is 14 days, prior to the formation of the primitive streak, morally significant?
- Is the acquisition of sentience in the fetus morally significant?
- Potential Human Being View. The two factors that are of moral significance are the actual status of the developing embryo and its potential for development.

Ethical issues at the beginning of life

'Life; a candle flame flickering in an open doorway.'

Buddhist Edict on Impermanence

Learning outcomes

After reading this chapter, you should be able to:
- Understand and evaluate the conservative view with respect to ethical issues at the beginning of life.
- Understand and evaluate the person or interest view with respect to ethical issues at the beginning of life.
- Understand and evaluate the view that treats the embryo or fetus as a member of the class of 'persons' with respect to ethical issues at the beginning of life.

In Chapter 9, we considered various accounts that have been offered about the beginning of life and the status of the embryo and fetus. We will now examine the implications of these different views for the cluster of ethical issues that arise at the beginning of life. Each view has implications for, for example, abortion, surrogacy, *in vitro* fertilisation, embryo research, embryo donation and use of fetal tissue. These are just examples of the issues that arise. However, a full understanding of the different views about the status of the embryo and fetus will enable the implications of these views to be worked out and applied to new problem areas. These will undoubtedly arise in the future with new advances in medical research. Although there might be ultimate disagreement in the views that are taken (see 3.2), it is important to operate with a view that can be held consistently over all these issues.

During the course of this discussion, we shall see that many of these questions are not solved by just considering the status of the fetus or embryo. In addition, other principles discussed in the first part of the book are also relevant.

10.1 THE CONSERVATIVE VIEW

The conservative view incorporates two claims. First is the claim that there is no morally significant dividing line in the development from fertilisation to the neonate stage. Second, since there is no morally significant dividing line, embryos and fetuses should be treated as we would treat human beings that have already been born. It is this second claim that makes the name 'conservative' appropriate since it is indicative of the opposition to abortion. Consequently, the only procedures that are permissible from the single-cell zygote onwards are those that are also accepted for human beings that have already been born.

10.1.1 Killing

A principle that we accept for human beings is that it is wrong to kill an innocent human being. Some people might also hold that it is wrong to kill any human beings, but for our purposes we can only consider the more restricted version of the principle since there is no question of the zygote onwards being anything other than innocent. Therefore, it would seem that if the zygote onwards is to be regarded as an innocent human being and it is wrong to kill innocent human beings then it is wrong to terminate the zygote's development through to birth. This principle is clearly relevant not only to the morality of abortion, but also to the permissibility of embryo research and further to the permissibility of creating embryos specifically for research.

ABORTION

According to the above account, abortion would be wrong. However, it is not quite this simple since we also need to consider the grounds for the requested abortion. For example, would we be committed to condemning abortion on this view if the abortion were necessary to save the mother's life? Both lives are innocent but it is not possible for both lives to continue. We have seen (see 7.2) that the Doctrine of the Double Effect has to be rejected so we cannot overcome this problem by arguing that our intention is to save the mother's life and the death of the fetus is just a foreseen but not intended consequence. Presumably, this sort of case would be analogous to killing in self-defence and would therefore be permissible if it was thought that this was justifiable. However, if killing in self-defence is also condemned so abortion to save the mother's life will also not be permitted. Therefore, the conservative view and the prohibition against killing innocent human beings do not lead to a clear-cut decision in this sort of case. In addition, an evaluation about the permissibility of killing in self-defence is also necessary.

It has also been argued that the conservative view does not necessarily imply the wrongness of abortions in other situations. Thomson[1] argues that the conservative position, that is essentially that the fetus has a right to life, does not imply that abortions are wrong. It must be recognised that the woman also has a right to determine what will happen to her body and it is not the case that the right to life will always take precedence over any other rights that are at issue. She draws an analogy with a case that involves two adult human beings. A famous violinist can only survive if he is plugged into your kidneys for nine months and you are kidnapped by the Society of Music Lovers to perform this function. Thomson argues that it would be generous if you agreed to stay wired up to the violinist but you are not obliged to.

The violinist's right to life does not take precedence over your right to determine what happens to your body.

Thomson is clearly adopting a deontological rather than a consequentialist approach (see 2.2 and 2.3) here, since one would suppose that a consequentialist analysis would yield the conclusion that you ought to allow the violinist to stay plugged into you kidneys. The consequences of disconnection will not only be the death of an individual but also the loss of a great deal of pleasure that this violinist can supposedly give. Hence, adoption of the conservative position results in different conclusions depending on whether it is considered from within a consequentialist or deontological framework.

Returning to Thomson's case, this is, at best, analogous to pregnancies started as a result of rape. The ground for claiming that the cases are analogous is that the conservative position accords the same status to the embryo and fetus that is accorded to human beings that have been born. However, it might be claimed that the analogy breaks down in at least one important respect. The fate of the violinist after the nine months is in no way the responsibility of the individual whose kidneys he has used, but this is not the case with a mother and her baby.

Singer[2] has extended Thomson's argument to cases of pregnancy that are commenced unintentionally. Here one has to suppose that an individual is visiting a hospital and presses the wrong lift button. She arrives at the floor where people go who have volunteered to be connected to those individuals who would not survive without this assistance. The same points made above about the rape case also apply here.

Clearly, the above three cases do not exhaust the reasons that can be advanced for an abortion. One of the central reasons for abortion requests is based on the grounds that the fetus is 'abnormal' in some way. In many of these cases there are existing human beings who are living with these conditions and it is not supposed to be justifiable to kill them. Hence, the conservative view leads to the same position with respect to fetuses that are found to be 'abnormal' in some way. Of course, if non-voluntary euthanasia (see 8.2.3) is thought to be justifiable for an individual then the conservative view would also sanction a similar case of non-voluntary euthanasia for the fetus.

Therefore, adopting the conservative view and the principle that it is wrong to kill innocent human beings entails that most abortions are wrong. However, those that are needed to save the mother's life might be justified. Also, if one accepts the sort of deontological analysis of rights proposed by Thomson, then abortions when the pregnancy has been commenced by rape or by accident might also be allowable. Abortions where the fetus is found to be suffering from a condition such as Down's syndrome or spina bifida would not be justifiable unless non-voluntary euthanasia could be justified in these cases.

CONTRACEPTION

The conservative view also implies that contraceptive methods that operate by preventing embryos implanting, such as the coil or 'morning after' pill, are wrong since effectively they are simply very early abortions. From the point of conception, the embryo is to be treated in the same way as an average adult member of the species, and hence this killing is unjustified.

EMBRYO RESEARCH

Embryo research is undertaken on embryos that have specifically been created for this purpose or from spare embryos resulting from infertility treatments such as *in vitro* fertilisation (IVF)[3]. Since the conservative view regards all stages from fertilisation onwards as having the same status as individuals of our species who have already been born, then embryo research is permitted since it inevitably ends in death. The same prohibition also applies to embryos that are specifically created for this purpose. Spare embryos will have to be frozen until there is the possibility of them being allowed to develop in the normal way.

10.1.2 Issues that do not involve killing

Surrogacy and *embryo donation to couples other than the generic parents* will not be prohibited on the conservative view of the status of the fetus, since the fetus is being allowed to mature to eventual birth. However, other principles that are relevant to these issues might lead to a different evaluation. In other words, although the conservative view does not prohibit these practices, they might be objectionable on other grounds and the conservative view does not preclude this. For example, prenatal adoption as the latter might be called might be objected to by the natural parents of the embryo on the grounds that only they wanted to bring their embryos to birth.

The use of fetal tissue is not prohibited on the conservative view. If it is considered acceptable to use organs from cadavers then it will be equally acceptable to use fetal tissue. However, it is an important issue, on the conservative view, to determine how the fetal tissue was obtained. If the fetal tissue was a result of a non-induced abortion then the use of fetal tissue is not prohibited. However, if the fetal tissue is obtained from an induced abortion then the issue is not clear cut on the conservative view. If the abortion was induced in order to obtain the fetal tissue, then this would not be justified on the conservative view. However, if this were done, further principles would need to be appealed to in order to determine what ought to be done with fetal tissue obtained from an abortion which would be prohibited on the conservative view.

In general, the conservative view involves treating embryos and fetuses in the same way as members of the human species that have already been born and the central thesis can be applied to all new procedures that become possible as the result of scientific advances. However, it has also become apparent that in many cases the conservative view alone is not sufficient to determine an answer to these ethical questions. Other principles need to be considered in conjunction with this view of the embryo or fetus.

10.2 THE PERSON OR INTEREST VIEW

The second view of the status of the fetus that we outlined in theChapter 9 is that held by Singer. This view, which we discussed in Chapter 3, holds that the fetus up to approximately 18 weeks does not possess interests since the nervous system is insufficiently developed for sentience to be possible. After this time, although it is sentient it is not a 'person' since it lacks rationality and awareness of it's existence over time, that is, it is not self-conscious.

10.2.1 Killing

ABORTION

In terms of the status of the fetus, the abortion of a pre-18–week fetus is comparable to killing something that is living but is not sentient. This, according to Singer, would raise no ethical issues since something that is living but not sentient can have no interests. Since Singer holds the consequentialist principle that the right action to perform is that action which maximises the interests of those affected then there is no fetal interest to enter into the calculation at this point. Singer writes:

> 'At least when carried out before 18 weeks, abortion is in itself morally neutral.'[4]

Hence, a consideration of the fetus would not prohibit abortion although other interests in the situation might count against it.

When we have a post-18–week fetus that is sentient, then the interests of the fetus have to be entered into the calculation along with the interests of all those others who are affected. According to Singer, sentient beings are replaceable, unlike 'persons', so if the loss of interest satisfaction of this fetus could be replaced by the creation, for example, of another fetus at a later date this would be an acceptable procedure.

CONTRACEPTION

All forms of contraception are permissible on this account since even if a post-fertilisation system is used, we only have a living being and not a sentient one.

EMBRYO RESEARCH

Embryo research and the creation of embryos specifically for research will be permissible on this view. It is also judged to be the right action to take if this is the best way to achieve such ends as improving techniques to deal with infertility. This would be the case if this view were coupled with the consequentialist principle that one should seek to maximise interest satisfaction.

10.2.2 Issues that do not involve killing

Surrogacy, embryo donation and the use of fetal tissue also not are prohibited on this view. They would not be prohibited since up to 18 weeks we have a living being who is not capable of feeling and hence has no interests. Whether these procedures are morally right or wrong will become clear if we couple this view with Singer's consequentialist thesis. If these procedures generate the maximisation of interest satisfaction then they are right. As Singer writes:

> 'I see nothing inherently wrong with more abortions, or with pregnancies being undertaken in order to provide fetal tissue, as long as the women involved are freely choosing to do this, and the additional abortions really do make some contribution to saving the lives of others.'[5]

10. 3 THE EMBRYO OR FETUS AS A MEMBER OF THE CLASS OF 'PERSONS'

The view that we support can be contrasted with the first two views in the following way. The 'person' view invites us to consider the *actual* status of the embryo or fetus.

At the early stages of pregnancy we just have a cluster of cells. Since these in themselves are not important then we do not have any ethical dilemma about, for example, aborting them. In contrast, the conservative view suggests that we ignore the actual status of the fetus or embryo and from fertilisation onwards accord it the same status as a human being who has already been born.

The view that we are proposing is that we consider *both* the actual developmental stage of the embryo or fetus and couple this with the recognition that this embryo is a member of a class of 'persons'. This latter term can be understood both from within the consequentialist framework that Singer adopts and also from the context of deontological theories. Kant argues that we must always treat rational beings as ends in themselves and not as means to other ends. He writes:

> *'Act in such a way that you always treat humanity, whether in your own person or in the person of any other, never simply as a means but always at the same time as an end.* [6]

One of the major implications of this is that it is indicative that there are limitations or constraints on what can be done in the pursuit of a good outcome. Rational beings cannot be used as a means towards the furtherance of a further end. Kant gives the example of someone who makes a false promise. Here we are using someone else as a means towards a further end that we desire.

Consideration of both the actual state of the embryo or fetus and recognition that it is a member of the class of 'persons', explains why we view issues such as embryo research, abortion and use of fetal tissue as *problem* issues. They would not be problematic if you just concentrated on the actual status of the development of the fetus and neither would they be problematic if the developing fetus is accorded the same status as other human beings. It is a view which explains the problematic nature of these issues but it does not, as with the other views, yield a solution to these problems in isolation from the consideration of additional principles.

10.3.1 Killing

On the conservative view, killing is generally condemned, and on the interest or person view, it is very often not prohibited and is often morally right. The view that we now consider provides much fewer clear-cut cases than either of the first two views and can perhaps be seen as a position midway between them. It is not as liberal as the person or interest view since it does not justify so many killings, but it provides justification for more killings than the conservative view. The problem becomes this: when are we justified in curtailing, by death, a member of the class of 'persons' whose actual status is not, as yet, that of a 'person'?

ABORTION

Within a deontological framework, we might consider that it is possible to treat the fetus as a means towards a further end in certain cases since it is only potentially an end-in-itself. For example, if the mother's life is at risk if the pregnancy continues then we have a conflict between the mother, who is an actual end-in-itself, and the fetus who is not. The fetus is biologically dependent on another individual who is an end-in-itself. Hence, clashes between a potential end-in-itself and an actual end-in-itself are necessarily very serious since the resolution of the clash, in the case of abortion, will lead to the death of the potential end-in-itself. However, when the mother's life is at risk, the actual end-in-itself ought to take priority over a potential end-in-itself.

If we have a pregnancy that occurred unintentionally, for example, either as a result of rape or by accident, then the autonomy of the woman if an abortion was denied would be overridden. She would be being treated as a means towards and end within a project that was not the result of her autonomous decision. Thus, abortion on these grounds appears to be permitted from a deontological perspective.

Within a deontological framework, it becomes important to consider the reasons advanced for the abortion. In the above case, the reasons were connected with how the pregnancy occurred. What about the case when a pregnancy is deliberately embarked upon with the intention of using the fetus as a means towards an end? This would not be allowable on this view since it would be denying the status of the fetus as an end-in-itself at the outset. This contrasts with the position taken in the 'person' view discussed earlier.

In the case of abortions that are undertaken for the sake of the fetus, for example, in the case of Down's syndrome or severe spina bifida, then these would be justifiable if euthanasia were considered to be justifiable for actual human beings with these conditions. The important point is that the abortion would be for the benefit of the fetus or embryo. It would be based on the claim that the fetus is a member of the class of ends-in-themselves. Although this position seems to flow naturally from the recognition of the autonomy of rational beings, Kant himself argues against suicide. He writes:

> *'If he does away with himself in order to escape from a painful situation, he is making use of a person merely as a means to maintain a tolerable state of affairs till the end of his life.*[7]

CONTRACEPTION

Clearly pre-fertilisation forms of contraception are permissible on this view but what about post-fertilisation systems? On the view under consideration we have to consider both the actual state of the embryo or fetus and take into account that it is a member of a class of 'persons'. At this very early stage of development, the autonomous decision of the mother would appear in most cases to render justifiable this form of contraception.

EMBRYO RESEARCH

Embryo research is undertaken on embryos that have been created specifically for this purpose or from spare embryos resulting from infertility treatments, such as *in vitro* fertilisation (IVF).[8] If we consider the actual status of the embryo up to 14 days we only have a cluster of cells. However, on the view that we are now considering, we also have to recognise that it is a member of a class of 'persons'. In Kantian terms, are we justified in using this cluster of cells as a means towards a further end or not?

Clearly, if we had an actual rather than a potential rational being Kant's answer would be in the negative. If we take the case of embryos that are specifically created for research, then this would appear to be condemned on this view since the fact of this being a member of the class of 'persons' is being denied from the point of fertilisation. An embryo created for research was always intended to be viewed as a means towards an end. These grounds for condemnation would only follow from within a deontological framework. Consequentialists would consider the possible beneficial outcomes of research in order to determine if it is justifiable. However, what about 'spare' embryos? These were created with a view to creating a 'person'. However, now that they are 'spare', how ought they to be treated? A consequentialist might very well argue at this point that if research were likely to yield beneficial outcomes then we would be justified in using the fetus as a means to an end at this stage of its development. It is debatable whether or not a deontological perspective would treat research on spare embryos as permissible. Even though they were originally created with a view to creating a 'person', can they now be viewed as a means to an end? Another factor that would immediately become relevant is the consideration of the views of the rational, autonomous individuals who donated their sperm and eggs for fertilisation. Since the embryo is not an actual end-in-itself it might be legitimate to use it as a means towards a further end if this is the autonomous decision of the donors.

The consideration of the donor, at least of the egg, presents another way of dealing with this problem. This view denies that there is any moral significance in whether the embryo was 'spare' or produced *in vitro* for research. Gerand[9] has argued that it is morally relevant to consider how the eggs were obtained. These eggs are obtained from women by first administering hormone stimulation therapy in order to obtain as many eggs as possible. Second, they are removed from women either by an ultrasound technique or by surgery in the form of a laparoscopy. Gerand argues that these techniques are a threat to women's autonomy. It is not possible for *informed* consent to be given since, for example, the long-term effects of hormone stimulation therapy are not fully understood. Also, the possible side-effects of the invasive procedures used to obtain the eggs are not always fully explained. She concludes that:

> '... *creating embryos for research should be questioned out of concern for the interests of the often ignored participants in the procedure: women.*'[10]

In Kantian terms, the woman's autonomy as a rational being is being undermined.

10.3.2 Issues that do not involve killing

Surrogacy and embryo donation are not prohibited on this view since the fetus are allowed to mature to eventual birth and 'personhood'. Other principles would have to be considered to determine whether or not these procedures were right but the view under consideration does not prohibit them.

The use of fetal tissue is prohibited on this view if the pregnancy was commenced with the sole purpose of utilising fetal tissue. This is because the status of the fetus as a potential 'person' would be being denied from the outset. The only intention was to treat this fetus as a means towards a further end. Fetal tissue obtained as a result of non-induced abortions or from abortions that are justified in accordance with this view could be used.

10.4 CONCLUSION

We have seen that when considering ethical problems at the beginning of life, the status of the embryo or fetus will not by itself yield solutions to these ethical problems

. The status of the fetus described above (10.3) appears to explain why it is that we view these issues as *problems.* Both the *actual* state of the fetus and its membership of the class of 'persons' has to be considered. If we combine this last view with a deontological approach then certain solutions to some of these problems are suggested.

As we have seen earlier in the book, there are certain reasons for favouring a deontological approach over a consequentialist one. Consequentialism leads to the downgrading of the moral significance of individuals. As Singer makes explicit in his *Principle of Equality* (see 6.2.1), it is interests that are to be treated equally and not individuals. In contrast, a deontological perspective recognises the importance and centrality of individuals within the field of morality.

LEARNING EXERCISES

1. An amniocentesis reveals that a woman is carrying a fetus that has Down's syndrome. She wants to have an abortion. Would an abortion be morally justifiable?
2. Ought research to be allowed on human embryos?

REFERENCES

1. Thomson, J.J. (1986) 'A Defence of Abortion'. In P. Singer (ed.) *Applied Ethics.* Oxford University Press, Oxford.
2. Singer, P. (1993) *Practical Ethics* (2nd edn). Cambridge University Press, Cambridge, p147.
3. Warnock, M. (1985) *A Question of Life: The Warnock Report on Human Fertilisation and Embryology.* Basil Blackwell, Oxford, p66.
4. Singer, *op. cit.*, p166.
5. Singer, *op. cit.*, p168.
6. Kant, I. 'Groundwork of the Metaphysic of Morals'. In H.J. Paton (1966) *The Moral Law.* Hutchinson University Library, London, p91.
7. *Ibid,* p91.
8. Warnock, *op. cit.*, p66.
9. Gerand, N. (1993) 'Creating embryos for research'. *Journal of Applied Philosophy,* **10**, 186.
10. *Ibid,* p186.

Key points

- The conservative view: There is no morally significant dividing line in the development from fertilisation onwards and embryos and fetuses should be treated as we treat human beings who have been born.
- It is wrong to kill an innocent human being.
- Abortion to save the mother's life.
- Abortions where the mother was raped.
- Abortions where the pregnancy was commenced unintentionally.
- Abortions where the fetus is 'abnormal'.
- The conservative view implies the wrongness of contraceptive methods that operate by preventing embryos implanting.
- The conservative view implies the moral unacceptability of embryo research.
- The conservative view does not prohibit surrogacy or embryo donation.
- The origin of the fetal tissue is relevant to whether or not the use of fetal tissue is allowable on the conservative view.
- The person or interest view. Approximately 18 weeks marks a morally significant dividing line between the sentient and non-sentient fetus.
- Abortion prior to 18 weeks is morally neutral.
- Abortion of post-18–week fetuses becomes a moral problem that is settled by calculating whether an abortion or no abortion would achieve the maximum amount of interest satisfaction.
- The person view will permit all forms of contraception.
- The person view will allow embryo research.
- The person view will not prohibit surrogacy, embryo donations and the use of fetal tissue.
- The embryo or fetus as a member of the class of 'persons'. Both the actual status of the fetus and its membership of the class of 'persons' needs to be considered.
- Killing. We are justified in curtailing, by death, a member of the class of 'persons' whose actual status is not, as yet, that of a 'person'.
- Abortion to save the mother's life is permitted.
- Abortion where the pregnancy was unintentional is permitted.
- Abortion would not be permitted when the pregnancy was undertaken with abortion as an aim.
- Abortion when the fetus is found to be 'abnormal' is only permitted if it is in the interests of that fetus.
- Contraception is morally acceptable.
- Embryo research is not permitted on embryos specifically created for this purpose. Further principles need to be appealed to to answer the question of whether or not embryo research should be permitted on 'spare' embryos.
- Surrogacy and embryo donation will not be prohibited.
- Whether the use of fetal tissue is justifiable on this view depends on the origin of the tissue.

Ethical issues at the end of life

'There should be no difference between the legality of switching on the machine and of switching it off. The law does not expect a doctor to place every dying patient on a life-support machine, only where there is hope of recovery and the facilities exist.' [1]

Learning outcomes

After reading this chapter, you should be able to:
- Apply, where relevant, the principles from the first part of the book to issues of whether to forgo treatment, prolong treatment or allow euthanasia.
- Understand the different issues that arise depending on whether you are dealing with autonomous individuals, those who have lost autonomy or those who have never reached a level of autonomy sufficient to take decisions in these areas.

11.1 THE PREMATURE BABY EXAMPLE

A baby born at 27 weeks' gestation suffered frequent collapses and required resuscitation and ventilator support. Ultrasound scans of her brain showed fluid-filled cavities where there should have been brain tissue. The view was taken that this tissue would not grow and the baby was likely to be blind, deaf, never able to sit up and have paralysis of both arms and legs. The baby would probably be able to feel pain but be unable to develop even limited intellectual abilities. If the baby suffers another collapse, ought she to be resuscitated and re-ventilated?

The above dilemma provides an illustration of a decision involving an individual who has never reached a level of autonomy sufficient to take their own decisions. Indeed, if the health care team's prognosis is correct, she will never achieve this capacity.

In this chapter, we consider dilemmas such as whether to forgo or prolong treatment and whether euthanasia is ever morally justifiable. These dilemmas are considered with respect to three different categories of individuals distinguished in the recent Stanley Report[2]. First we have decisions involving individuals who have decision-making capacity or who have executed advance directives about such decisions. Second, there are those who have lost this capacity and have not executed an advance directive. Finally, there are decisions involving those who have never achieved decision-making capacity as in the above example. The discussion will be related to the different concepts of death discussed in Chapter 9 and will highlight the relevance of the principles discussed in Section 1 of the book.

11.2 DECISIONS INVOLVING INDIVIDUALS WHO HAVE DECISION-MAKING CAPACITY OR WHO HAVE LEFT ADVANCE DIRECTIVES

In these cases, one principle that is immediately relevant is that of the Principle of Autonomy (see 4.1). Here we have individuals who have the capacity to think and make decisions. Ought their decisions always to take priority over other considerations?

11.2.1 Decisions to forgo treatment

If we take a deontological justification of the Principle of Autonomy (see 4.2.2), then the wishes of an individual who decides to refuse treatment are paramount. If this decision is based on sufficient information about the treatment and alternative treatments, then the decision ought to be respected.

A consequentialist justification of the Principle of Autonomy might not appear to generate the same conclusion (see 6.2). Here, recognition of the Principle of Autonomy will be justified if this recognition leads to outcomes being as good as possible. It might be felt by the health care team that the individual's decision to forgo this treatment will not lead to the best outcome. However, the conflict between the individual's autonomy and what might be considered to be the best outcome by the health care team can be resolved. What must be remembered is that what counts as the best outcome is the result of an evaluative decision. From the individual's perspective, the best outcome will be what he or she considers will result from the refusal of treatment. This might not be viewed as the best outcome from the perspective of the health care team. Consequently, if the consequentialist justification of the Principle of Autonomy is coupled with the individual's assessment of what is the best outcome, then the individual's decision ought to be respected.

11.2.2 Requests for life-prolonging treatment

These are sometimes not so easy to deal with as the above. For example, there are scarce resources and hence there might not be enough resources to grant every request for life-prolonging treatment. If this is the case, how ought we to decide between competing claims? What is a just way to allocate limited health care resources?

In terms of principles, the Principle of Autonomy is clearly relevant since we are supposing that the autonomous decision of the individual is that life-prolonging treatment is wanted. However, a Principle of Justice is needed to consider the rival claims of individuals if resources are limited.

We have already rejected in Section 1 of the book a consequentialist justification of the Principle of Justice (see page 00). This is because such a concept ignores the competing claims of *individuals* and instead concentrates on how much of a certain benefit will be achieved by different allocations. The maximisation of interest satisfaction or quality adjusted life years is what is of value rather than a consideration of the equitable distribution of these 'benefits' *between* individuals.

A deontological justification of the Principle of Justice (see page 00) concentrates on the competing *needs* of individuals rather than concentrating on the maximisation of a certain outcome. This principle should be applied at both the macro- and microallocation level. In other words, we need first at the macroallocation level a just distribution of money to health care expenditure as opposed to, for example, defence, education and transport. We also need at this level a just distribution of resources within the health care budget. Second, at the microallocation level, we have the question of a just distribution between individuals. Clearly, the microallocation level is highly dependent on decisions taken at the macroallocation level since that determines the availability of treatments. Therefore, conflicts between the Principle of Autonomy and the Principle of Justice should be solved by a consideration of the relative needs of the separate individuals and not by a consideration of what would yield the maximisation of something like interest satisfaction.

Of course, some requests for life-prolonging treatment do not require us to consider the competing claims of other individuals. When there is not a scarcity of treatments, ought the individual's autonomous decision to be respected? Three points mentioned in the Stanley Report[2] suggest that the individual's autonomous decision is not necessarily paramount. For example, if the health care team consider that the treatment will be futile in the sense of not achieving the desired physiological change, ought the treatment to be given? Second, if the treatment involves pain disproportionate to the benefit that is hoped for, ought the treatment to be given? Finally, if a member of the health care team has a conscientious objection to the requested treatment, ought the treatment to be given?

These first two points appear to throw doubt on whether the original decision was really autonomous. To make an autonomous decision, it is necessary to have information about the treatment and alternative treatments. If the treatment will definitely not achieve the desired physiological change, then it would be irrational to request it. The second point above is liable to lead to paternalistic interventions in individuals' lives. Benefits and pains are a matter for the *individual* to assess and will be reflected in the individual's autonomous decision. To allow for the overriding of an individual's autonomy on these grounds is to open the way for paternalistic infringements of individuals' autonomy.

In connection with the final point made in the Stanley Report, this could be overcome by referring the individual to another doctor. Therefore, these three points do not appear to provide grounds for overriding an individual's autonomy.

11.2.3 Requests for euthanasia

These will be cases of voluntary euthanasia (see 8.2.3) since the individual is assumed to possess the required level of competence necessary to make this request. The decision to die is a reflection of the individual's autonomy and if it has been carefully considered (see 8.2.3) and is not a transitory wish, then it ought to be respected. However, the autonomy of the person to whom the request is made must also be considered. If they hold, for example, that life is sacred then they should not be required to adhere to this request. Referral to another doctor must remain an option for the individual who requests euthanasia.

With all the above issues, it should perhaps be emphasised that the reliance on advance directives about what should be done is not so reliable as the consideration of a request given contemporaneously with the decision to be taken.

11.3 DECISIONS INVOLVING INDIVIDUALS WHO HAVE LOST THE DECISION-MAKING CAPACITY

At this stage of our discussion, the accounts of the concepts of death given in Chapter 9 become relevant. One such group of individuals falling within this class are those in a persistent vegetative state. Another group are those who have temporarily lost this decision-making capacity.

11.3.1 Decisions to forgo treatment

With respect to the person view and the capacity for a consciousness view about death, those in PVS are classed as being dead. Hence, it is inappropriate to talk about a decision to forgo treatment. With the other views, we have an individual who is alive.

Since this individual cannot be consulted, who ought to be consulted and who ought to take the decision to forgo treatment? Presumably, we should make the decision, as with the class of cases already discussed in this chapter, that would most reflect the individual's wishes if he or she could communicate. Hence consultation with close relatives and friends to determine as much as possible about this individual is required. The basis of this claim would be to arrive at a decision which is as close as possible to the decision that the individual would him- or herself have made if this was still possible for him or her.

This knowledge of the individual would include, as highlighted in the fifth group of views in 9.2.1, a consideration of their spiritual beliefs which might well determine how they would have viewed a decision to forgo treatment.

It has been argued that the decision to forgo treatment must be shared.

> 'In the case of the PVS patient, the determination of irreversibility can only be made by doctors ... the determination of continued treatment as futile and thus optional, should be a shared judgement.' [4]

This judgement should be shared, it is argued, between the doctor and the individual's surrogate. This should surely be extended to include other members of the health care team. For example, it is often the nurse who is most closely involved with an individual and their family. Expertise in clinical diagnosis does not automatically confer expertise in ethical decision making (see 1.2). Decisions to forgo treatment will be easier if it is generally publicised that this is an option.

In the case of individuals who have only temporarily lost their decision-making capacity, then if possible this decision ought to be deferred until this capacity has been regained. If this is not possible, then a decision which reflects as closely as possible their autonomous wishes is the one to aim for.

11.3.2 Decisions to institute life-prolonging treatment

It might be supposed that those individuals in a PVS have no self-regarding interests. Indeed, the Stanley Report asserts this[3]. The report goes on to state that from this it follows that there are no patient-based reasons for continuing life-sustaining treatments. However, a knowledge of the individual's previous values and ideals is relevant when considering the continuation of life-sustaining treatments.

For example, the individual might have held that life itself is sacred even if the life is no longer capable of consciousness. Hence, although there has not been an explicit directive about what they would wish done if they were in this situation, their previous value system provides an indication of their wishes. The individual was previously an autonomous agent and hence this factor needs to be reflected in the decision. However, it is true that an individual in a PVS has no *actual* interests at this present time since they have lost all powers of cognition and sentience. Therefore, this means that their views, based on the knowledge of their previous value system, can be overridden. The actual interests of the relatives and the health care team are also relevant. Also, as with the cases in 11.2.2, scarce resources make the Principle of Justice a relevant principle for consideration. What is the fairest way of distributing resources if there is a shortage of, for example, intensive care facilities?

This decision should not be taken on a consequentialist basis. It should not be taken on the basis of what would lead to the maximisation of a particular outcome but should instead be based on the competing needs of the individuals as discussed in 11.2.2 and 6.3.

With respect to individuals who have temporarily lost the capacity to make decisions, the points made in 11.2 will be the ones that are relevant. The only difference will be that an informed judgement will have to be made about what this individual would want if they still had the decision-making capacity.

Euthanasia

These would be cases of non-voluntary euthanasia (see 8.2.3) since the individual is not in a position to communicate their views about the continuation of their life. The Stanley Report distinguishes forgoing treatment and active euthanasia:

> *'Intervention with the primary intention of causing death (as distinguished from forgoing treatment that is deemed appropriate) has no place in the treatment of permanently incapacitated patients. However, vigorous treatment to relieve pain and suffering may well be justified, even if these interventions lead to an earlier death.'[5]*

This quotation exhibits an implicit reliance on both the *acts and omissions doctrine* and the *Doctrine of the Double Effect* (see 7.1 and 7.2). In the second sentence there is an assumption that there is a difference between what one aims at as opposed to what is foreseen but is not primarily intended. One is aiming at the relief of pain although the foreseen consequences of this course of treatment are the earlier death of the individual. However, as we argued in 7.2, this distinction is not viable. Hence, the same considerations apply here as in the section above on forgoing treatment. Clearly, the quoted paragraph is not referring to those individuals in a PVS since they are not in pain or suffering.

The first sentence includes the implicit assumption that there is a difference between acts and omissions (see page 00). Omitting treatment is distinguished from an active intervention to cause death. However, as we argued on page 00, where a conscious decision has been taken to bring about the death of an individual then there is no moral difference between bringing this about by a positive act or omission. The omission in this sort of case is more appropriately described as an *act* of omission (see 7.4).

In the case of individuals in a PVS, it would appear that the same points could be made about non-voluntary euthanasia as for decisions to forgo treatment as described in 11.3.1.

11.4 DECISIONS INVOLVING THOSE WHO HAVE NEVER ACHIEVED DECISION-MAKING CAPACITY

An example of this sort of case is the 'premature baby example' described at the beginning of the chapter. In this example, we are assuming that the baby, if she lived, would never be able to achieve decision-making capacity. However, there are also cases where it might be supposed that the baby does have the potential to develop decision-making capacity in the future. It will be important to bear this distinction in mind since it has implications for the relevance of the Principle of Autonomy. As discussed in 11.3, the individual's previous autonomy was relevant to the decision and here the individual's future autonomy is relevant. As was argued in 10.3 , *both* the actual state and future state are relevant.

11.4.1 Decisions to forgo treatment

If we take the person view of death advocated by Rachels, then, since the baby in our example will never be capable of having a biographical life, it is permissible to forgo treatment. The baby will be able to feel pain and suffer but not develop any of the intellectual abilities associated with being a 'person'. They will never be in a position to take autonomous decisions and have, in Rachel's terms, a biographical life. Hence, since it is biographical lives that are of value, according to Rachels, rather than merely biological lives, then it is justifiable from this point of view to forgo treatment. Also, there is a positive reason for forgoing treatment. If we continue treatment then the pain that this baby is suffering will continue.

However, if we have a case where it is supposed that the baby will be capable of sustaining a biographical life, then to forgo treatment will be denying this benefit. It will be denying something that is essential for this baby's development into an autonomous individual. This would, on this view, be a much more serious matter than in the 'premature baby example'.

11.4.2 Decisions to institute life-prolonging treatment

In the 'premature baby example', life-prolonging treatment had been given but the question arose of whether it should be given again. We have a baby who is in pain and does not have any prospect of becoming an autonomous agent. Prolongation of the baby's suffering is not in the baby's interest. Also, the baby is not in a position to value their own life and never will be in this position. From this perspective, then, there would appear to be no grounds to institute life-prolonging treatment. As well as the interests of the baby, we also have the interests of the family and health care team to consider. However, the central concern is still the suffering of the baby which would continue if life-prolonging treatment is continued or re-instituted.

When this case is also viewed in the context of other cases where there might be a demand for scarce life-prolonging treatments, then these treatments ought to be allocated to those who have a better prognosis than the baby in our example. Life-prolonging treatment ought to be given to those babies who have the chance of sustaining biographical lives in the future.

11.4.3 Euthanasia

These cases of non-voluntary euthanasia would appear to raise the same issues as those connected with forgoing treatment (see11.4.1). If death is intended, then there is no moral difference between forgoing treatment to achieve this end and active euthanasia (see 7.1 and 7.2).

In the case of non-voluntary euthanasia involving individuals who will become autonomous, we have to insure that the decision is taken in their best interests since we shall be denying them the realisation of this state.

LEARNING EXERCISES

1. Are we morally justified in forgoing treatment where the individual is in a persistent vegetative state?
2. Do autonomous individuals have a right to life-prolonging treatment if they request it?

REFERENCES

1. Dimond, B. (1990) *Legal Aspects of Nursing,*Chapter 16, p230, Citing Kennedy, I. (1977: Criminal Law Report, p443). Prentice Hall, UK.
2. Stanley, J.M. (1992) 'Developing guidelines for decisions to forgo life-prolonging medical treatment'. *Journal of Medical Ethics,* **18**, Supplement.
3. *Ibid*, p11.
4. Mitchell, K.R., Kerridge, I.H. and Lovat, T.J. (1993) 'Medical futility, treatment withdrawal and the persistent vegetative state'. *Journal of Medical Ethics,* **19**, 74–5.
5. Stanley, *op. cit.*, p11.

Key points
- The decision of an autonomous individual to forgo treatment ought to be respected.
- Requests for life-prolonging treatment by autonomous individuals should be respected if there is no competition for resources. If there is a scarcity of treatments then the relative needs of the competing individuals should be considered.
- Requests for euthanasia by autonomous individuals ought to be respected.
- Where an individual is no longer autonomous, decisions to forgo treatment should reflect as closely as possible what it is considered that that individual would have wanted.
- Where an individual is no longer autonomous, decisions to prolong treatment should take account of their previous wishes and their actual present state.

- If non-voluntary euthanasia is thought appropriate, there is no moral difference between bringing this about by a positive act or by omission.
- Where an individual has never achieved autonomy, decisions to forgo treatment, prolong treatment or perform non-voluntary euthanasia must be based on both the actual state of the individual and the potential future state of that individual .

CHAPTER 12

Ethical issues in information exchange: confidentiality, informed consent, truth telling

'Anyone who thinks that disclosure of confidential information is morally justified, or even mandatory in some circumstances, bears a burden of proof. While this approach requires a balancing of conflicting duties, it also establishes a structure of moral reasoning and justification.' [1]

Learning outcomes

After reading this chapter, you should be able to:
- Discuss the moral and legal rationales for maintaining confidentiality of information.
- Identify exceptions to the duty of confidentiality.
- Discuss the moral justification for obtaining informed consent to treatment.
- Critically discuss the moral principles which may justify or refute disclosure of dire information to patients.
- Explain how information exchange between health professionals and patients/clients should be addressed within the context of a therapeutic relationship.

12.1 CONFIDENTIALITY

From both moral and legal perspectives, the rationales for maintaining the confidentiality of information relating to individuals, both verbal and in records, are extremely powerful and compelling. Strong justifications must be made for breaking this duty, which should only occur in exceptional situations. How can confidentiality be justified, both morally and legally? From a legal perspective Dimond[2] cites three major duties from which arise the duty of confidentiality:
- The duty of care arising from common law and following from the health care professional/consumer relationship (see Chapter 15).

- Implied duties arising under the contract of employment, wherein an employee has responsibilities to an employer to maintain confidentiality of information gained in the process of work. For medical practitioners and nurses, these duties are clearly delineated in codes of professional conduct.
- A duty based on equity which requires information related in confidence to be maintained confidential. This applies in the absence of legally enforceable contracts or relationships between the parties.

From the perspective of professional ethics, the precept that health care professionals should maintain the information divulged to them by individuals in strict confidence, is enshrined in the professional codes of conduct for nursing, midwifery and health visiting and also in medicine. In the latter, the principle is explicitly stated in the Hippocratic Oath:

'... *whatever ... I see or hear in the life of men which ought not to be spoken of abroad, I will not divulge'.* (See Appendix B.)

Although the British Medical Association recognises that exceptions to the duty of confidentiality can arise, the World Medical Association maintains that it is an absolute duty of professional conduct which continues to apply after the death of a patient. In the case of nursing, midwifery and health visiting, Clause 9 of the UKCC Code of Professional Conduct requires that practitioners in the exercise of their professional accountability, shall:

'... *respect confidential information obtained in the course of professional practice, and refrain from disclosing such information without the consent of the patient/client ... except where disclosure is required by the law, or by order of the court, or in the public interest'.*[3]

In addition to this emphasis placed on confidentiality in Clause 9 of the Code of Professional Conduct, the UKCC[4] have provided more detailed guidelines in the form of an advisory paper, containing a framework to assist individual professional judgement, recognising that complex situations and dilemmas can arise in practice (see Appendix).

The nature, components and virtues inherent in the caring relationship which exists between health professionals and recipients of care, lies at the heart of the duty to respect the confidentiality of information. Caring relationships are built on trust, worth, dignity and endowed with compassion and positive mutual regard[5]. The information divulged within the context of this relationship is vital to enable effective, high-quality care to be provided. It can be regarded as privileged, in the sense that it is obtained entirely by virtue of the nature of the professional relationship and is not at the level of that exchanged in normal, everyday social interaction. It may cover personal, social, financial and medical areas of the individual's life. Information concerning details of the diagnosis, prognosis, symptoms suffered and aspects of treatment are the most obvious areas covered by the duty of confidentiality. The Patients Charter[6] emphasises the confidentiality of such information in relation to citizens' rights, stressing that information about the progress of treatment will only be divulged subject to the individual's wishes. The onus is firmly placed on the health professional to ascertain precisely what the views of individuals are concerning what they wish others to know, and to respect these wishes.

12.1.2 Justification for confidentiality

Confidentiality is a moral, professional and legal duty. How may it be justified on moral grounds? A deontological justification is based on the principle of respect for the autonomy of the individual (see 4.2.2). The recognition of the intrinsic value of autonomy is also essential for the survival of relationships with others, and vital in the context of the professional relationship, where individual patients/clients are to be recognised as ends in themselves (see 4.4). Marshall[7] views the exercise of autonomous control concerning information about thoughts, feelings and personal information to be revealed or concealed as important aspects of selfhood which must be respected. Respect for autonomy can also be justified on consequentialist grounds (see 4.2.1). Respect for autonomy also encompasses respect for privacy; that is, an individual's autonomous choice in choosing what to disclose or conceal about self. This autonomous right of individuals to have information about themselves kept private is emphasised in the UKCC[4] framework (elaboration of Clause 9 of the Professional Code of Conduct), which requires practitioners to consider the devastating personal, social and legal consequences which could follow unauthorised disclosure of information. Considerations of non-maleficence are also relevant here for the health professional who 'ought to do no harm' (see 5.1).

Preserving confidentiality can also be justified on the consequentialist grounds that it will maximise benefits to the individuals who will be able to openly divulge to the health practitioner information which is vital to their treatment and other aspects of care. Confidentiality is then justified morally, in that the best possible outcomes in health care are achieved for the individual (see 2.2).

12.1.3 Exceptions

Exceptionally, situations can arise in which confidentiality of information can be breached either in the individuals or public interest. From a moral viewpoint respect for autonomy may not be justified where there is a serious risk of harm to others (see 4.2.1).

Exceptions to the duty to maintain confidentiality include the following:

WITH THE INDIVIDUAL'S CONSENT
Power to authorise disclosure of information to the media, relatives or other parties rests with the individual or their legal advisor. The responsibility lies with the health professional to ascertain from the recipients of care on every occasion what may be divulged either verbally or by telephone and to whom, with his or her express consent.

IN THE INDIVIDUAL'S INTEREST
It is clearly in the individual's interest that disclosure of information takes place between the health professionals concerned with care. Not only will this facilitate effective co-ordination of care, but it will minimise the risks of errors or harm. Access to the medical/nursing records is vital for health care professionals. If this were not the case, consider what the risks of accidental injury could be if the physiotherapist had no information concerning:
• individuals suffering from a neurological disorder who were vulnerable to sudden

onset epileptic fits;
- unstable diabetics, vulnerable to hypoglycaemic attacks when exercising.

COURT ORDERS

A court of justice does not recognise that health professionals possess special privileges to withhold information. To do so could result in prosecution as an accessory after the fact in criminal proceedings.

STATUTORY REQUIREMENTS

Disclosure of confidential information can be required by the law in circumstances covered by the Prevention of Terrorism Act, Misuse of Drugs Act, Road Traffic Act, Abortion Act, Public Health Act, Police and Criminal Evidence Acts (see Dimond[2, 8] for case law).

THE PUBLIC INTEREST

The situation can arise where a health professional must breach confidentiality to protect the health and safety of others. A controversial and difficult area, the dilemmas are well illustrated in relation to AIDS-infected health care workers. The UKCC in relation to such health workers attending occupational health departments, states:

> '... it is accepted that there will be rare occasions in which professional
> practitioners in occupational health, faced with an HIV-positive practitioner
> engaged in exposure-prone procedures who is not complying with specialist advice
> to change her or his area of practice, may deem it necessary to communicate
> information concerning the practitioners' HIV status to the appropriate medical
> practitioner of the employing authority in confidence and to the individual's
> professional regulatory body'.[9]

In conclusion, the duty of confidentiality is fundamental to codes of professional practice, and the maintenance of trust in therapeutic relationships. Strong justifications must be made if it breached; exceptions when this may be necessary are listed above. Two case studies (see 12.3) illustrate situations where breaches of confidentiality occurred, when a fatal diagnosis was discussed with relatives but not the recipients of care. The implications of this are discussed in 2.3.

12.2 INFORMED CONSENT

> 'To be given a clear explanation of any treatment proposed including any risks
> and any alternative, before you decide whether you will agree to treatment.'[10]

Informed consent is defined as:

> '... a voluntary, uncoerced decision, made by a sufficiently competent or
> autonomous person, on the basis of adequate information and deliberation, to
> accept or to reject some proposed course of action which will affect him/her'.[11]

As is evident from this definition and the statement cited above, from the Patients Charter, the key issues related to informed consent are encapsulated in the use of terms such as 'agree', 'accept' and reject'. Decision making here, is placed firmly within the competent patient/clients control, but do they all wish to assume responsibility for decisions related to treatment? What are the justifications for informed consent? How can we define 'adequate information'?

The moral justification for obtaining consent to treatment is based on respect for the autonomy of rational agents, the treatment of individuals as ends in themselves (see 4.2.2). Respect for autonomy can also be justified on consequentialist grounds (see 4.2.1). From a legal perspective, freedom from interferences is viewed as a basic human right, and a mature, rational individual may choose whether or not to submit to treatment. If consent is not obtained, the patient/client could have ground to bring legal charges of trespass, assault or battery. In addition, failure to provide adequate information can constitute a breach of duty of care, and the risk of legal actions for negligence being brought against the health professional.[2, 12] An important consideration here, is that obtaining satisfactory consent then places the weighing of risks on the patient/client, protecting the health professional from civil actions if problems occur later.

In the past, objections to obtaining informed consent from patients have arisen from paternalistic concerns that imparting information about medical procedures and possible risks, associated with the role of complex terminology, could cause considerable anxiety and alarm in addition to problems of comprehension. Such paternalistic considerations of beneficence and non-maleficence could justify individuals being spared concerns about their impending treatment. The counter argument here is that giving them information, particularly that which is appropriate and comprehensible, does not necessarily impair their rationality and ability to exercise judgement. A health professional who is sensitive and skilled in communication can discover what the individual already knows, and needs to know, together with the terminology and language which will ensure that information is understood. It is vital that information giving is appropriately timed and that further opportunities are created for follow up discussions to clarify issues and eliminate misunderstandings.

A number of case study reports have suggested that some individuals do not wish to take an active role in decision making in relation to aspects of their medical treatment and care[13, 14] (see16.5.3). Respect for autonomy requires that patients' wishes are consulted and the extent to which they wish to be involved in decision making clarified. Surrender of autonomy by waiver is morally acceptable, if an individual's wishes have been respected and they have intentionally, willingly agreed to a plan of treatment proposed by the doctor or other health professional; that is, the decision has been autonomously delegated.

Occasionally, the situation can arise where a rational, competent adult who has requested information, received and fully comprehended it, decides to refuse any medical treatment, for example, blood transfusions, chemotherapy, surgery, which may be life saving. This poses a considerable dilemma for health professionals. Should the individual's autonomy in decision making be respected? For medical and nursing practitioners bound by a duty of care, who wish to act with beneficence and non-maleficence, ethical and legal principles are in conflict. In this situation, respect for the autonomy of rational agents takes precedence. Furthermore, the right of a competent adult to refuse treatment is also enshrined in law[2].

12.2.1 Types and components of consent

Three forms of consent to treatment are recognised as valid in a legal context: implied, oral and written. However, implied consent, suggested by behavioural responses, that is, attendance at an outpatient clinic, does not imply agreement to anything other than superficial medical examination. Expressed consents, either orally or in writing, are necessary in the context of other clinical situations. For minor therapeutic procedures, for example, blood sampling, oral consent is normally used, but Knight[12] suggests that this should be obtained in the presence of an unbiased third party. In the case of blood sampling, apart from a diagnostic test for AIDS, consent to give blood for testing implies consent to all those tests which the medical practitioner considers are in the individual's interest (beneficence). The UKCC [9] have advised practitioners that they expose themselves to the possibility of litigation or professional misconduct if they obtain or co-operate in obtaining blood samples for AIDS testing without consent. However, it is acknowledged that rare and exceptional circumstances might arise where unconsented testing could take place legitimately. Strong justification (on beneficent, non-maleficent grounds) would have to be made in these exceptional cases, that the diagnostic procedure was again in the individual's best interest.

Express consent in writing, which constitutes the best form of evidence, is required for all other major diagnostic procedures, surgical or medical treatments, including general anaesthetics, which involve varying degrees of risk; the consent that is given must relate to a specific procedure/operation only.

Five elements can be discerned which informed consent should cover in relation to information given to the patient:
- The prognosis of their condition if left untreated.
- The range of treatment options available.
- The discomforts and risks associated with each option.
- Side-effects, whether the treatment is successful or not.
- Purposes and potential benefits of the treatment.

Since an effective, responsible decision cannot occur without acquiring the knowledge necessary to make an informed choice, consent must be obtained after a 'reasonable' explanation covering the points cited above.

The question then arises, what is 'reasonable' information? In the UK conclusions regarding this have been deduced following the *Sidaway Case* in 1985, which involved an appeal to the House of Lords. This case concerned a medical practitioner's alleged negligence and liability in respect of failure to warn an individual of the risks associated with an operation on the spinal column. The information adjured by the judges as 'reasonable' was that accepted as proper by a responsible body of medical opinion, that is, by peer review. This paternalistic self-regulatory approach (the 'Bolam' Test), is not considered entirely satisfactory by many, who consider that lay public opinion on what is reasonable should also be considered in deciding what constitutes the most reasonable information with which to make an informed decision. The need for information to be honest and accurate is vital in relation to informed consent. The issue of truth telling in information exchange is discussed in 12.3.

12.2.2 Obtaining consent: impaired autonomy

Competent adults (over 16 years of age) provide consent for their medical treatment. For individuals below this age, consent is sought from either parent or guardian, unless an emergency arises (Family Law Reform Act 1969). However, children under 16 years can give consent if judged by a medical practitioner to have sufficient maturity of mind and comprehension, but in practice every effort should be made to involve the parents in such a decision.

In situations where autonomy of thought or will is impaired, can consent be obtained? Precisely how much autonomy does an individual have to possess to be respected as an autonomous agent[11]? The array of ethical and legal case study data on decision making in situations of impaired autonomy is vast and the reader is referred to specialised texts for a detailed consideration of these cases. Suffice it to say, beneficent interventions can be justified by medical practitioners, for example, in situations of impaired consciousness or the sterilisation of mentally handicapped minors[8]. In the case of psychiatric illness, impaired thought (delusions) can co-exist with a rational understanding related to physical illness and the need for treatment. Here, the situation is sometimes not clear-cut particularly with individuals who oscillate between periods of rationality and seriously impaired comprehension. Consent to treatment provisions for long- and short-term detained individuals and those categorised as 'informal' are covered by the Mental Health Act 1983.

12.2.3 Living wills

In certain states within the US the concept of a 'living will' may be upheld by the law. As originally developed this is a document which enables 'individuals, while competent, to inform family members and health providers of their wishes regarding the use of life-sustaining treatment when death is imminent'[15]. Modified definitions include 'instructions to withdraw or withhold life sustaining procedures when those serve no purpose except to artificially delay the moment of death';[16] also 'withholding or withdrawing any measure that would through artificial means prolong life in a terminally ill person unable to decide at the time'[17]. The US laws related to these documents vary, but most state that individuals enacting a living will must have attained the age of consent (normally 18 years) and be competent at the time. Witnesses are required who, in many instances, must not be potential heirs. Requirements to be met before carrying out instructions contained in living wills include independent medical confirmation that the individual's condition is terminal; medical practitioners who enact the living will are released from criminal liability.

Strong justification for the living will is based on respect for the autonomy of individuals to self-determination, a principle which has also received support from provisions in the AHA Patient's Bill of Rights. Opponents of this proposal base their counter arguments on the uncertainty of medical prognoses, invalidation of informed consent and that euthanasia could be condoned[18].

12.3 TRUTH TELLING

'The most striking contradiction of our civilisation is the fundamental reverence for truth which we profess, and the thoroughgoing disregard for it which we practice.' [19]

Historically, the duty of truthfulness has not been prominent in medical therapeutic relationships:

> *'Deception is completely moral when it is used for the benefit of the patient'.*[20]

A variety of reasons may account for the difficulties which health professionals encounter in telling individuals bad news about their diagnosis, treatment and prognosis. Beneficence, non-maleficence and paternalism may be primary considerations, but poor communication skills, lack of knowledge, uncertainty, fear of blame from colleagues, patients, families, attitudes to death and identification with recipients of care, may be all contributory. In this section of Chapter 12, truth telling is considered in relation to giving individuals dire information about their diagnosis, treatment and prognosis, notably in relation to mortal illness, death and dying. From a moral perspective, can beneficence ever justify lying? On what grounds can this be refuted? How can conflicting ethical principles be reconciled or ordered, and what are their implications for decision making?

12.3.1 A case for deception?

Health professionals have duties to benefit the welfare of their patients and above all to do no harm (see 5.1, 5.2). A general justification for not telling individuals the truth about a mortal diagnosis or prognosis is that to do so would cause great suffering, depression and the removal of hope or 'fighting spirit', which could impair the quality of their remaining weeks or months of life (see 2.1). Important questions here are, would deception maximise benefits and produce the best consequences? In these situations, who is best able to judge what is of benefit – the recipients of care, the doctor, or some other health professional? In the previous discussion on informed consent to treatment, the duty to ensure that the individual is informed of risks and side-effects of therapy was described. However, in relation to terminal illness, a mortal diagnosis or prognosis, information can be withheld from the individual if it is deemed in their best interests not to know, that is, if there is risk of harm. This is known as therapeutic privilege and requires the careful exercise of clinical judgement[8]. The following case studies exemplify situations where therapeutic privilege and considerations of beneficence have been applied in specific instances.

CASE STUDY I

A young married couple have been involved in a major road traffic accident and are brought into casualty, unconscious and suffering from multiple injuries. The husband, who was driving the family car, subsequently dies from serious head injuries. Following major surgery, his wife is ventilated in the intensive care unit, where her condition is critical due to hypovolaemic shock. After 48 hours, she regains consciousness and is able to breath spontaneously without mechanical ventilation, but her condition remains very serious. She asks the medical and nursing staff what has happened to her husband. Concerned that the bad news could, at this stage, reduce her chances of survival they decide to withhold the truth and tell her he is extremely ill until, in their judgement, she is able to cope with the information without adverse effects. Relatives concur with this decision.

CASE STUDY 2

A middle-aged man with a lengthy past medical history of gastrointestinal problems is admitted to hospital suffering from weight loss and abdominal pain. Investigations confirm the presence of a gut carcinoma which has metastasised to the liver, giving him a life expectancy of three to six months. Over many years the medical consultant has come to know his patient extremely well and is aware that his particular hopes, wishes, joys and aspirations in his life plan include competing in the local bowls championship (imminent) and the birth of his first grandchild. In view of this, and with the agreement of the individual's family, the doctor decides not to tell the patient of his diagnosis. After securing effective pain control he allows him to leave hospital under the impression that his health is not beyond recovery. He returns to work for a short time, competes in and wins the bowls championship and lives to nurse his new granddaughter. Three months later he is readmitted to hospital, in a terminal condition, where he dies peacefully, never knowing his diagnosis.

CASE STUDY 3 (EXTRAPOLATED FROM HIGGS[21] AND DUNBAR[22])

An elderly lady suffering from chest pain and breathing difficulties is admitted to hospital for investigation. A cancerous tumour of the lung is discovered, which has metastasised to distant organs giving her a life expectancy, at most, of six months. The surgeon discusses the diagnosis and prognosis with her husband and family, who ask him not to tell her that she has cancer; 'nothing can be done and it is better that she does not know'. Over the subsequent five months, her condition deteriorates and she becomes very distressed and anxious about the lack of information concerning her condition. Eventually, her GP, a family friend, tells her the truth at her own request. She dies peacefully, without anxiety, a few days later.

Cases such as these also highlight the conflicts which can occur between the principles of beneficence, non-maleficence and autonomy in decision making. In addition, the breach of confidentiality and emergence of other interests in the cases are important aspects, which are considered further below.

Other arguments which can be advanced to justify non-disclosure of information and deception are that health professionals do not possess, or cannot know, the absolute truth and therefore cannot communicate this. Even if the truth could be communicated, another frequently cited reason for not telling the truth is that, in general, recipients of care could not understand it. Medical conditions and their associated terminology are complex, when asked to define commonly used medical terms a number of past surveys have shown that individuals knowledge and understanding is inadequate.[23, 24]

A further reason advanced for not telling the truth concerning diagnosis and prognosis is that individuals do not wish to know 'bad news'. This assumption can also be questioned in terms of its applicability to the general population.

12.3.2 Refuting deception

THERAPEUTIC RELATIONSHIPS

Information exchange occurs within the context of the therapeutic relationship between the individual and health professional, which is based on trust. Bok[25] suggests that there is a moral presumption against deception, lies and non-disclosure of information in therapeutic relationships, since trust can be destroyed by deception.

Indeed, deception can be viewed as an unacceptable form of paternalism in which the autonomy of a rational individual is denied. It can be argued that the duty of veracity is intrinsic to therapeutic relationships, which are also rooted in other duties of respect, fidelity and confidentiality which obviate deceit. Questions about the nature of therapeutic relationships arise from the breaches of confidentiality and trust evident in case studies 2 and 3. The principle of veracity did not form the core of the value systems of the medical practitioners concerned with these cases, with the exception of the GP in case 3, who knew the recipient of care as a person, and was in touch with her value systems, priorities and, presumably, her life plans. It would have been a fairly straightforward matter for the surgeon in case 3, to have contacted the GP, to have ascertained to what extent she could have coped with the diagnosis. Such an approach would not have breached professional confidentiality (see 12.3).

Commenting on factors which affect the notions of trust and veracity in doctor-patient relationships, Dunbar [22] suggests that doctors may engage in deception because they do not wish to recognise the individual who is terminal as a vulnerable person. Since the medical condition is terminal and cannot be alleviated, this may be perceived as personal failure. In addition, health professionals may not be able to cope with reminders of their own mortality, a further reason for evasion within the relationship.

Dunbar[22] and Higgs[21] have commented on the different approaches to truth telling inherent in care of individuals suffering from cancer and AIDS, noting that the truth is always told about diagnosis and treatment to the latter. Reasons which may explain these differences reside ultimately in the nature of the therapeutic relationship. AIDS is a condition which cannot be cured; in the absence of curative intervention, do the qualities, virtues and strengths inherent in the therapeutic relationship become the most important aspect of treatment?

ETHICAL PRINCIPLES IN CONFLICT: AUTONOMY TAKES PRECEDENCE

The major refutation of arguments justifying deception on the grounds of beneficence (cases 2 and 3) arises from considerations of respect for autonomy. Respect for the principle of autonomy, and rights to self-determination of rational agents (see 2.1 and 2.3) would require that in such situations, for example, cases 2 and 3, individuals should be told the truth about their diagnosis, treatment and prognosis and be enable to remain in control over the remaining period of their lives. Furthermore, from a deontological perspective 'the rightness of telling the truth is intrinsic to truth telling itself, and is not dependent on truth telling resulting in good consequences' (see 2.3). Respect for the autonomy of rational agents could also be justified from a consequentialist stance, since Mill considered that respect for autonomy (equated with liberty, see 4.2), could be justified as producing the best outcomes as long as harm to others did not occur.

In case 2, appeals for beneficent, paternal deception are justified on the basis that the doctor had particular insight into the personal values, aspirations and life plans of the individual. However, we cannot know what the autonomous decision of the individual would have been had he been given an opportunity to know the truth. In the light of such knowledge he may have re-ordered priorities and plans very differently to those perceived and proscribed by paternalistic, medical practice. Collins[26], in attempting to justify beneficent paternalism recounts similar cases of deception producing the best outcomes as judged by doctors; and also describes cases where telling the truth was followed by a rapid decline and premature demise of the individual. However, the consideration that telling the truth could be harmful in individual cases, is not a justification for general policies of non-disclosure, which would deny the autonomy of many.

It is frequently argued that beneficent deception can be justified on the grounds of minimising suffering and harm. Review of case 3 demonstrates that, in fact, exactly the reverse may happen. Deception once engaged may have to be sustained over a long time period, during which anxiety, depression and stress can be engendered by uncertainty. Not only may these adversely affect the individual, but the need for continued lying may erode the quality of the relationship within the family, causing guilt and remorse for relatives during future grieving.

The duty of confidentiality was breached by medical practitioners in cases 2 and 3, who informed the relatives of the individual's diagnosis and prognosis without their authorisation for disclosure. Again, this infringed autonomy and violated the trust inherent in a caring relationship. Childress[27] and Dunbar[22] emphasised that the primary responsibility of health professionals is to the individual; the interests of the family are to be regarded as secondary considerations in situations such as this. An interesting point to emerge from case 3 is that the family, having been told first of the individual's fatal condition, suggested deception apparently for beneficent reasons. Dunbar[22] suggests that other motives may have been influential, for example, self-interest or an inability to cope with the reality of death and dying.

Gillon[11] and Childress[27] have argued that, in relation to truth telling, respect for the principle of autonomy takes precedence over considerations of beneficence and non-maleficence. Are there any exceptions to this? Dunbar[22] considers that concealment of diagnostic information may be justified if the risk of suicide is high. (Presumably this risk would be weighed on the basis of past medical history and current psychological status?) Higgs[28] suggests that the situation exemplified in case 1 would justify setting aside the duty of veracity, since considerations of beneficence, non-maleficence and the patient's continued survival are paramount.

IS THE TRUTH KNOWN OR UNDERSTOOD?

An argument which has been used to justify non-disclosure of information in truth telling is that the absolute truth can never be known. Diagnostic and prognostic information can only be couched in terms of probabilities and non-certainties. Childress[27] points out the fundamental confusion in this argument, which fails to distinguish between philosophical debate concerning the nature of truth and the moral issues/responsibility for telling the truth to someone, that is, stating honestly what is believed to be true on the basis of the available facts. The argument that non-disclosure is justified on the basis that individuals cannot understand medical information can also be refuted. The onus here is placed firmly on the communication skills of the health professional in relating technical details in a comprehensible way. If plumbers and electricians can disseminate technical information in terms which are understood by the lay public, why cannot health professionals?

WISHES TO KNOW OR NOT?

Contemporary perspectives on information exchange in relation to truth telling suggest that disclosure of diagnostic information is now more common, although differences do exist between cultures. For example, thirty years ago 90% of medical practitioners in the USA did not divulge a diagnosis of cancer to individuals; a tenet which has undergone almost a total reverse (see 16.6.2). In contrast, in Japan it is still not obligatory for doctors to divulge a diagnosis of cancer, a medical practice which has received backing from a high court ruling. In Japan, cancer carries a considerable social stigma.

Possible reasons for changing perspectives on diagnostic disclosure in the US and Europe include changes in public perception about cancer, the rise of consumerism, an emphasis on active consumer participation in care and in the US and fears of lawsuits for malpractice.[14, 27] Two justifications underpin contemporary views. The first is deontological, suggesting that disclosure is in the individual's best interests to permit the exercise of autonomy and that they have rights to know. A second reason is that informed patients are able to participate more effectively in their care, and it is therefore in their interests to do so. Childress[27] comments that an approach which grants individuals access to information based on a consideration of their interests remains paternalistic and fails to address the issue of rights.

While many recipients of care wish to have information about their diagnosis, prognosis and treatment, others may request non-disclosure or, having been informed, do not wish to be involved in decision making[13, 14, 29]. In respecting autonomy, it is vital that the health professional clarifies with the individual, in a skilled and sensitive way, precisely how much they already know and how much information they wish to have. Information should be given as it is requested, in language which is comprehensible. It is important to consider that information needs of individuals change over time; an initial view or reaction may not be the final view and may change. A realistic amount of time must be devoted to such discussions with the recipients of care, together with opportunities for follow up. If they refuse to accept information and make it clear that they do not wish to know dire consequences, as long as their wishes have been consulted and they have exerted an autonomous right in refusing, respect for autonomy has been maintained. Since this option does not harm others, it should be respected. Rights to know must be respected as much as rights not to know. Occasionally situations arise where a request for non-disclosure of diagnostic information is made, but risks to others must be considered. For example, disclosure of a diagnosis of AIDS, or other serious infection, could be justified on consequentialist grounds as necessary to minimise harm to others who could become infected and whose autonomy must also be considered.

It is not uncommon for individuals who have been told that they are dying to engage in denial behaviour, which may be an initial reaction to 'bad news' or can be intermittent and mark a stage in their progress towards final acceptance[30]. Childress[27] considers that we have rights to deny, which must be respected as much as rights to know. It is vital that health professionals can recognise emotional responses to approaching death and can adjust informational support accordingly.

In conclusion, respect for autonomy provides a strong justification for truth telling, where patients wish to receive information. Byrne[31] comments that communication according to a 'general formula', which suggests that we should all be told the unvarnished truth whether we wish it or not, violates the requirements of moral relationships and fidelity. Respect for autonomy, requires that after consultation of an individual's wishes, rights to know are respected as much as rights not to know.

LEARNING EXERCISES

1. Discuss the ethical issues which can arise in information exchange between health professionals and patients.
2. Discuss the nature, components and virtues in a caring relationship which affect the exchange of diagnostic and prognostic information.
3. Discuss how you would obtain informed consent in relation to (a) patient participation in a randomised, controlled clinical trial; and (b) a patient who requires chemotherapy for malignant disease. What ethical principles should inform your conduct?
4. Deception is justified if used for the patient's benefit. Discuss.
5. Respect for autonomy takes precedence over beneficence in therapeutic interventions. Discuss.

REFERENCES

1. Beauchamp,T.L., Childress, J.F. (1979) *Principles of Biomedical Ethics.* Oxford University Press, New York.
2. Dimond, B. (1993) *Patients Rights, Responsibilities and the Nurse.* Quay Publishing, UK.
3. UKCC (1992) *Code of Professional Conduct for the Nurse, Midwife and Health Visitor.* UKCC, London.
4. UKCC (1987) *Confidentiality: An Elaboration of Clause 9 of the Second Edition of the UKCC Code of Conduct for the Nurse, Midwife and Health Visitor.* UKCC, London.
5. Leininger, M. 'Historic and epistemologic dimensions of care and caring'. In *Knowledge About Care and Caring* (1990) (Eds. J. Stevenson,T. Tripp–Reimer, T.) American Academy of Nursing. Kansas, USA.
6. Department of Health (1992) *The Patient's Charter: A Summary.* HMSO, London, UK.
7. Marshall, S.E. (1988) 'Public bodies, private selves.' *Journal of Applied Philosophy.* 5(2):147–158.
8. Dimond, B. (1990) *Legal Aspects of Nursing.* Prentice-Hall, UK.
9. UKCC (1994) *Acquired Immune Deficiency Syndrome and Human Immunodeficiency Virus Infection.* Position Statement; Annexe 1 to Registrars Letter. 4/94. UKCC, London, UK.
10. Department of Health,*op. cit.*
11. Gillon, R. (1986) *Philosophical Medical Ethics.* John Wiley, UK.
12. Knight, B. (1989) *Legal Aspects of Medical Practical.* Churchill Livingstone, UK.
13. Waterworth, S., Luker, H.A. (1990) 'Reluctant collaborators: do patients want to be involved in decisions concerning care? *Journal of Advanced Nursing,* 15:971–976.
14. Biley, F. (1990) }Some determinants that affect patient participation in decision makinbg about nursing care'. *Journal of Advanced Nursing,* 17:414–421.
15. Mathews, K. (1986) 'Living Wills: do nurses and physicians have them?' *American Journal of Nursing,* 8:26–29.
16. Creighton, H. (1986) *Law Every Nurse Should Know.* W.B. Saunders, Philadelphia, USA.
17. Anderson, G.C. (1986) 'Living Wills: do nurses and physicians have them?' *American Journal of Nursing,* 86:271–275.
18. Ney, A. (1989) 'Living Wills: The Ethical Dilemmas'. Critical Care, *Nurse* 9(8):20–41.
19. Stefansson, V. (1977) Cited in 'Quotations for Our Time', *Truth* pp499–502. Ed. L.Peter, Methuen, London.
20. Leslie, A. (1954) 'Ethics and practice of placebo therapy.' *American Journal of Medicine,* 16: 854–862.
21. Higgs, R. (1982) 'Truth at last: a case of obstructed death.' *Journal of Medical Ethics,* 8:48–50.

22. Dunbar, S. (1990) An obstructed death and medical ethics. Journal of Medical Ethics, **16**:83–87.
23. Smeltzer, C. (1980).'Hypertensive patients' understanding about terminology.' *Clinical Ethics in Critical Care*, **9**(3):498–502.
24. Pearson, J. (1982) 'Bodily perceptions in surgical patients.' *British Medical Journal*, **284**:1545–1546.
25. Bok, S. (1978) *Lying: Moral Choice in Public and Private Life*. Pantheon Books, New York.
26. Collins, J. (1981) 'Should doctors tell the truth?' In *Biomedical Ethics*, pp64–67. Eds. A.Thomas, J.S. Zembaty, McGraw-Hill, USA.
27. Childress, J. (1982) *Who Should Decide?* Oxford University Press, UK.
28. Higgs, R. (1990) 'An obstructed death and medical ethics.' *Journal of Medical Ethics*, **16**:90–92.
29. McIntosh, J. (1976) 'Patients' awareness and desire for information about diagnosed but undisclosed malignant disease.' *The Lancet*, August 7, **300**.
30. Kübler-Ross, E. (1969) *On Death and Dying*. Macmillan Press, New York.
31. Byrne, P. (1990) 'Comments on an obstructed death'. *Journal of Medical Ethics*, **16**:88–89.

Key points

- The duty of confidentiality. Non-disclosure of confidential information by health professionals arising from duties of care, equity and those implied by contract.
- Deontology. Certain prima facie duties such as truth telling, non-maleficence, justice, beneficence are morally obligatory.
- The Principle of Autonomy. In certain areas an individual has a right to be self-governing.
- Consequentialism. There is one ultimate moral aim, that outcomes be as good as possible.
- Informed consent. Voluntary agreement by an adequately informed, autonomous person, to investigation or treatment.
- Strong paternalism. Limiting or denying freedom of choice to a competent person capable of making an autonomous decision.
- The Principal of Beneficence. The well-being or benefit of the individual ought to be promoted.
- The Principle of Non-maleficence. One ought to do no harm.

CHAPTER 13

Ethical issues in health care research

'Science goes forward only through new ideas and creative thought.' [1]

Learning outcomes

After reading this chapter, you should be able to:
- Identify the ethical principles inherent in health-care research.
- Discuss how research workers can act to promote the well-being and benefit of participants.
- Explain how the autonomy of participants may be respected in research protocols.
- Critically discuss the concept of 'fair equitable research'.
- Describe how the current roles of ethical committees may be developed and improved.

13.1 INTRODUCTION

Few would argue that progress in biomedical research has not benefited humankind during the last century. From this has arisen the knowledge which has dramatically improved not only the quality and duration of life, but also the morbidity and mortality associated with some diseases previously known to cause profound suffering, or to obliterate entire populations. Although its benefits are acknowledged, the nature and evolution of experimentation on human subjects has always raised ethical questions. These must be subjected to critical appraisal by the health care professional engaged in research and by the consumer who may be approached as a potential participant. In the main, these questions relate to principles of autonomy, justice, beneficence and non-maleficence, which have been considered in Chapters 4–6 and are reviewed here in the context of health care research.

A number of professional bodies have evolved their own guidelines for health care professionals engaged in researc; in the UK these are the Royal College of Nursing,

British Medical Association and General Medical Council in the UK. Concern about research involving human subjects at an international level led the World Medical Association to develop guidelines enshrined in the1975 'Declaration of Helsinki'. These encapsulate key ethical precepts of autonomy, beneficence, non-maleficence and also consequentialist calculations, evident in the extract below:

> *'Every biomedical research project involving human subjects should be preceded by a careful assessment of predictable risks in comparison with foreseeable benefits to the subject or to others. Concern for the interests of the subject must always prevail over the interests of science and society.*[2]

The Declaration of Helsinki not only identified important parameters within which biomedical research could take place, but also made a crucial distinction between non-therapeutic and therapeutic research. The former includes research on healthy volunteers and individuals for whom 'experimental design is not related to their illness'. Here, the participants do not benefit from new knowledge generated by the investigation but others may do so at a later stage. In contrast, therapeutic research involves recipients of care for whom a definite relationship exists between the research and their illness. A possibility of direct benefits may accrue to them, ranging from the relief of unpleasant symptoms, to a cure for their disease, or to an increase in the duration and quality of life.

13.2 BENEFICENCE

The principle of beneficence (see 5.2) requires that health care professionals engaged in research act to promote the well-being and benefit of participants. In the research context, this encompasses prevention from exposure to undue risks or situations for which participants are unprepared. It is also essential to ensure that information gained in data collection does not have negative repercussions on individuals. For example, participants in a quality assurance survey might make critical observations about the institution in which they work. Assurances should be given concerning the confidentiality of their responses (see 12.1).

Considerations of beneficence require researchers to perform a consequentialist justification (see 5.2) for their investigation, by assessing the potential benefits versus risks for participants. As is the case with many consequentialist approaches, these calculations are not easy to do as benefits and risks may not be quantifiable. The benefits, which may vary in accordance with the therapeutic or non-therapeutic nature of the research, could include relief of symptoms, improved quality of life, cure of disease, enhanced knowledge of self, improved self-esteem and monetary or material gains. Against this must be weighed the risks of unwanted, harmful side-effects, loss of privacy and possible psychological distress arising from disclosure of personal information.

Important questions here are: to what extent are risks known and how can they be quantified? Can research workers be objective in risk assessment? In the UK, risks associated with new drugs are evaluated by prior testing in animal models, but these are not always extrapolated to human subjects with absolute certainty, only probability in terms of their predictive value. The quantification of risk is also rather crude, but negligible risk can be defined as 'less than that run in everyday life'. Minimal risk has been defined as 'risks anticipated in the proposed research are not greater, considering probability and magnitude, than those ordinarily encountered in daily life, or during the performance of routine, physical or psychological examinations or tests'[3]. These definitions cannot be accepted uncritically, since they assume that the risks associated with everyday life are known and quantifiable. A high degree of subjectivity can also be involved in their interpretation. Clearly, risks exceeding 'minimal' are normally unacceptable in research.

Principles of beneficence, justice and respect for the participants' autonomy require benefits, risks and consequentialist justifications associated with research proposals to be scrutinised in external review, by an unbiased committee. Appraisal by an independent ethical committee, whose principle remit is to protect the autonomy and rights of potential participants, is an essential safeguard. Above all, benefits and risks must be evaluated by autonomous, informed participants after due reflection. They may weigh benefits and risks in an entirely different way to the research investigator (informed consent, see 12.2).

Professional codes of conduct enshrine the principles of beneficence and non-maleficence, by requiring health care personnel to act positively for the well-being and benefit of their patients or clients and 'to do no harm'[4]. Upon such principles are founded the therapeutic relationship of trust between nurses, doctors and the recipients of care, the consumers who assume that their best interests are always considered first. In the research context, a different relationship operates, and Gillon[5] has made the point that research subjects may erroneously assume that the usual, beneficent therapeutic concerns of health care professionals will apply to them, but this is not possible within the definition of non-therapeutic research. Similarly, the assumption made by individuals, that doctors will expose them to risks only in the light of a favourable cost/benefit analysis is not again the case in non-therapeutic research, where the benefits are accrued by others. These distinctions, between the normal therapeutic relationship and that operating in the research context, must be clarified with potential participants at the outset.

13.3 NON-MALEFICENCE

'Above all, do no harm' (see 5.2) is a central tenet of research; the exposure of participants to harm, physical or psychological, is entirely unacceptable. It is incumbent on research workers and ethical committees to ascertain that the safeguards which ensure harm does not occur are securely in place. These include requirements for research workers to be appropriately qualified, for new drugs to have satisfied the Committee on the Safety of Medicines and for investigations to be terminated at the earliest indication of untoward effects, in so far as these are known. The latter are obvious where physical symptoms or pathological changes are measurable. Less obvious are the psychological sequence of intrusive questions on personal subjects, that is, those eliciting information about experiences and feelings in relation to an illness (which may have been traumatic) or painful relationships. The requirement for non-maleficence makes it necessary for health care researchers to incorporate sensitivity in their approach and to consider the effects of questions on their subjects. Debriefing sessions provided after data collection is complete, can permit participants to ask questions and to clarify any anxiety-evoking issues that may have arisen.

13.4 AUTONOMY

'In any research on human beings, each potential subject must be adequately informed of the aims, methods, anticipated benefits and potential hazards of the study and the discomfort it may entail. He or she should be informed that he or she is at liberty to abstain from participation in the study, and that he or she is free to withdraw his or her consent to participation at any time. The doctor should then obtain the subject's freely given informed consent, preferably in writing.' [2]

Principles of autonomy – 'self rule' – can be justified, as discussed in 4.1, from both a utilitarian and a deontological perspective. Individuals are autonomous agents with rights to self-determination. Respect for autonomy and individual rights requires that patients/clients/healthy volunteers have the right to decide whether or not to participate in a research study, free from coercion and without prejudice. Some interpretations by Local Health Authorities of the Patients' Charter[6] now specifically state that patients have rights to be asked whether or not they wish to take part in medical research and to know that any decision will not affect the care received.

However, coercion can be implicit and unintentional or explicit. Polit and Hungler[7] suggest that the nature of the relationship between the nurse or doctor and recipient of care can be unequal in terms of power. If the health professional is perceived by the potential subject to be in a position of authority and control, then this could involve a coercive element in relation to participation in a research study. This point should be considered carefully by all health professionals engaged in research, whose intentions are beneficent. Mild, explicit coercion may arise in situations where financial payments are offered to the economically or socially disadvantaged, as inducements to participate in research studies. Recent reports in the UK press have expressed concern at the recruitment of unemployed individuals to drug trials run by pharmaceutical companies who may not be operating within strict, ethical guidelines.

Respect for autonomy requires participants to make informed, voluntary decisions about participation in research (see12.2). The deontological, Kantian perspective requires individuals to 'act in such a way that you always treat humanity, whether in your own person or in the person of any other, never simply as a means, but always at the same time as an end'.(see 4.2.2) As noted in Chapter 4, as rational agents, other people as well as ourselves can set ends and make rational choices. In relation to research participation, it is only permissible to use someone as a means to an end if they share that end and consent to it. Without informed consent, the participant is used as a means, a violation of their autonomy. **Table 13.1** summarises the range of points which should be considered in obtaining informed consent. Information should be presented verbally and in writing, allowing time for questions. In order for risks and benefits to be carefully weighed, adequate time must be allowed for reflection. It is critical that the information is understood or consent is not valid. Language used should be clear, concise and avoid medical jargon. The views of lay persons on ethical committees can be extremely useful in advising on the formulation of comprehensible information. Accurate documentation of consent, usually by the researcher and participant signing a form designed for the purpose, is necessary, and in some cases the presence of a third, independent party is desirable. Although variation in practices is evident, some ethical committees do not require written consent if the research is minimal in risk, non-invasive and non-intrusive, for example, some types of survey research, involving postal questionnaires, where the respondents have complete freedom in deciding whether to participate or not.

Some ethnographic research methods require non disclosure of information in order to avoid bias. Data collection may be covert or entirely concealed. Examples of this type of research include observations of nursing behaviour or practices and the observation of mother-child interaction through a two-way mirror in a hospital clinic waiting room. This type of research is usually justified on the grounds that the risks are negligible, rights to privacy are not breached, and there are considerable benefits to science and society.

The randomised, controlled clinical trial also presents ethical problems in terms of design and disclosure. Here, subjects may be allocated to experimental or placebo groups to evaluate a new type of medical treatment. It is vital that informed consent is obtained before randomisation and that participants fully understand that they may be given a placebo. Instances have arisen where individuals have been entered into clinical trials without their knowledge, believing they were given a type of treatment which the medical practitioner judged appropriate for their illness and its stage of development. Clearly, frank deception in which information is withheld or false information provided is morally unacceptable, and is a violation of autonomy and the subject's right to make an informed decision. It can also expose the health care professional to litigation proceedings. Situations may arise where a nurse discovers that either informed consent has not been obtained from an individual entered into a research trial or that the information given has been misunderstood. In such cases it is the nurse's responsibility to notify the medical researcher and request that information is given which is comprehended. If a refusal to tell the participant is elicited then the nurse has little choice but to report the incident to a manager and to disclose the information to the individual him or herself. In the context, the nurse is acting as an advocate, a role fraught with difficulties (see page 00). Failure to obtain consent to research or to give the necessary information, could render the researcher liable to legal action.

Table 13.1 Components of informed consent

- Explanations concerning the purpose of the investigation, its duration and the commitment required from participants.
- Type of information to be obtained during the study, including special procedures.
- Uses of information.
- Information on potential, foreseeable risks and, if appropriate, unforeseeable risks.
- Potential benefits to participants.
- Emphasis that consent is voluntary.
- Rights to withdraw.
- Details of alternative treatments that exist (therapeutic research).
- Assurances on confidentiality.
- Points of access should participants require information at any time.

Research in vulnerable groups

Ethical committees must implement additional policies and procedures to protect the rights of individuals whose autonomy of thought, will or action is impaired, or who are particularly vulnerable to side-effects by virtue of their medical condition. Problems which arise in cases of impaired autonomy include failure to comprehend and weigh up information, or to be physically incapable of signing a consent form. Into this category are placed minors, the mentally handicapped and those suffering from neurological or mental illness. Pregnancy may render a woman more vulnerable to physical and psychological side-effects and, in addition, the status and well-being of the fetus must also be considered.

From both ethical and legal perspectives, minors cannot give informed consent, which is obtained from parents or guardians. In conjunction with this, written consent demonstrating respect for self-determination can, however, be obtained from a minor who has sufficient maturity. Parents cannot give valid consent to research procedures not in the child's best interests or where significant risk exists[8]. The Declaration of Helsinki states that non-therapeutic research requires volunteers to make a free choice, after due comprehension, analysis and reflection on information received. This requires the autonomous deliberation of rational agents, which excludes minors. It is the principal reason why some suggest that children should not be involved in non-therapeutic research, which offers them no prospect of benefit. Counter arguments to this are that it is the level of risk posed by the research which is morally relevant – not its nature – and the consequentialist view that benefits to other children are relevant to moral deliberation. In therapeutic research, which offers the prospect of benefit, different considerations apply to the participation of minors. Here, the level of risk must be carefully weighed and guidelines to aid risk assessment have been developed by the British Paediatric Association[9]. From a legal perspective, Dimond[8] comments that where the child cannot receive personal benefit from research, there can be no justification for submitting to even minor levels of risk.

13.5 JUSTICE

The Principle of Justice, that equals ought to be treated equally (see 6.1) also applies to the participation of subjects in research studies.

Fair, equitable treatment, in the context of research, is interpreted by Polit and Hungler[7] to include the following:

- Non-discrimination in selection based on research criteria.
- Equitable sharing of risks and benefits between participants.
- Non-prejudicial treatment for those who refuse to participate or withdraw during the investigation.
- Provision of access to research personnel to clarify any matter.
- Immediate assistance if harmful side-effects occur.
- Provision of debriefing sessions to allow participants to discuss issues that may have arisen during or after the research study.
- Honouring of financial agreements.
- Consistency in adherence to research procedures agreed when informed consent is obtained.

Rights to privacy must also be considered in relation to the Principle of Justice. Ensuring anonymity or employing other confidentiality procedures can ensure that privacy is safeguarded. Specifically, confidentiality of information can be ensured by:
- Requiring research assistants to sign confidentiality agreements.
- Use of coding numbers for subjects.
- Restricting access to identifying information and destroying it as soon as possible.
- Maintaining locked files and complete avoidance of computer logging of identifying information.
- Reporting research findings in such a way that individuals cannot be identified – sparing descriptions should be used in case studies.

13.6 ETHICAL COMMITTEES

In order to protect the autonomy and rights of potential participants, the ethical dimensions of research studies on human subjects should be subject to independent evaluation. Most hospitals, clinical research centres and academic institutions have ethical committees for such purposes, which operate through formal procedures and protocols. In general, these aim to ensure safety in monitoring freedom from harm or exploitation, equitable selection and to guarantee rights to privacy and anonymity. In addition, confidentiality must be maintained and informed consent safeguarded (see 12.1 and 12.2).

Ethical committee practices do vary within and between countries. In the UK concern has been expressed about their independent, idiosyncratic function and diversity in operation, which could result in some not reaching acceptable standards, risking exposure of research subjects to unsafe practices. Their diversity is also a check on the prospect of valuable, multicentre research[10, 11]. Although professional bodies have issued guidelines, these may be interpreted variably and ethics committees may discriminate on which aspects they will follow or avoid. For example, they may not elect a lay member as Chair or Vice-Chair, due to feelings that such a person is not credible in medical knowledge.

Current weaknesses in the UK system of ethical review noted by Foster[11] include:
- The proliferation of committees within and outside the NHS, without central registering mechanisms or legal framework.
- An absence of mechanisms for monitoring standards in relation to function.
- No accreditation body.
- Variability in constitution, procedures, protocols.

Particular strengths of the UK system appear to be the shift of ethical committees towards a Kantian perspective, emphasising the unacceptability of using participants as 'ends'. Foster[11] notes their growing recognition of important moral distinctions, for example, between not harming a person (physically, psychologically or in damaging their interests) and that of wrongdoing, by violation of their autonomy. Other strengths are seen to be the positive benefits in insisting that health care professionals disclose full, clear information and their freedom from bias due to peer pressure on decision making.

13.6.1 Improving the system

Current concerns about the operation of ethical committees could be alleviated by providing guidelines which stipulate minimum standards of practice, in relation to structures, procedures and methods for approval of therapeutic/non-therapeutic research. The European Commission[12] has produced guidelines itemising specific points upon which a researcher is required to seek the opinion of an independent committee. These include approaches used in recruitment, obtaining informed consent, scientific rationale for the research protocol and the justification of risks weighed against benefits for participants. Other approaches to optimise and standardise the operation of ethical committees could include the formation of self regulatory bodies and the introduction of training programmes for members[10].

In summary, the participation of human subjects in research raises ethical questions related to autonomy, beneficence, non-maleficence and justice. High standards of professional practice in research can be assured by implementing the strategies which ensure autonomy is respected, harm prevented and the rights of the individual maintained. Accountability for these rests with ethical committees, professional bodies and all health care professionals engaged in therapeutic and non-therapeutic research (see 15.1).

LEARNING EXERCISES

1. What is 'informed consent'? Discuss how it may be obtained from potential participants in a research study.
2. Discus the components of an ethical research study design.
3. Impaired autonomy: discuss the issues in relation to therapeutic and non-therapeutic research.
4. Respect for autonomy: how may this be preserved in relation to research participation?
5. Beneficence and non-maleficence: discuss in relation to professional roles in the research process.

REFERENCES

1. Bernard, C . (1865). *An Introduction to the Study of Experimental Medicine.* Copley-Greene, H. (trns)(1957). Dover Publications, New York, USA.
2. *Declaration of Helsinki: 'Recommendations Guiding Physicians in Biomedical Research Involving Human Subjects'.* Adopted by the 18th World Medical Assembly in 1964 and revised by the 29th World Medical Assembly in Tokyo, 1975.
3. US Department of Health and Human Services (1981). 'Final Regulations for Amending Basic NHS Policy for the Protection of Human Research Subjects.' *Federal Register,* **46**(16):8366–88.
4. UKCC (1992). *Code of Professional Conduct for the Nurse, Midwife and Health Visitor* (3rd end). UKCC, London.
5. Gillon, R. (1986). *Philosophical Medical Ethics.* John Wiley, Chichester, UK.
6. Department of Health (1992). *The Patient's Charter: A Summary.* HMSO, London, UK.
7. Polit, D.F. and Hungler, B.P. (1991). *Nursing Research: Principles and Methods* (4th end). J B Lippincott, Phildelphia, USA.
8. Dimond, B. (1993). *Patients Rights, Responsibilities and the Nurse.* Quay Publishing, UK.

9. British Paediatric Association Guidelines (1980). 'Guidelines to Aid Ethical Committees Considering Research Involving Children'. *Archives of Diseases of Childhood*, **55**(1):75–7.
10. Neuberger, J. (1992). *Ethics Committees in the United Kingdom*. Kings Fund Publication, London.
11. Foster, C.G. (1993). 'The Development and Future of Research Ethics Committees in Britain'. In *Choices and Decisions in Health Care*. Ed. Grubb, A. John Wiley, Chichester, UK, pp161–81.
12. 'Guidelines on Good Clinical Practice for Trials on Medicinal Products in the European Community'. 111/3976/88-EN. European Committee for Proprietary Medicinal Products, July 1991.

FURTHER READING

Department of Health (1991). *Local Research Ethics Committees*. HS.6(91)5. Department of Health: London.

Dimond, B. (1990). *Legal Aspects of Nursing*. Prentice Hall, London.

Faulder, C. (1985). *Whose Body is it? The Troubling Issue of Informed Consent*. Virago Press, London.

Freedman, B. (1975). 'A Moral Theory of Informed Consent'. *Hastings Centre Report*, **5**(4), 32–9.

Gaylin, W. (1982). 'The Incompetence of Children: No Longer All or None'. *Hastings Centre Report*. *Independent.*, 19th October 1993.

GMC (1981). *Local Ethics Committees*. General Medical Council., London.

Kant, I. (1981). *Grounding of the Metaphysics of Morals*. Ed. Ellington, J.W. Hackett, Indianapolis.

Ramsey, P. (1970). *The Patient as a Person*. Yale University Press, New Haven.

Royal College of Physicians (1990). *Research on Patients*. Royal College of Physicians, London.

Rumbold, G. (1993). *Ethics in Nursing Practice* (2nd edn). Baillière Tindall, London.

Veatch, R.M. (1981). *A Theory of Medical Ethics*. Basic Books, New York.

Key points

- The Principle of Autonomy. In certain areas an individual has a right to be self-governing.
- The Principle of Beneficence. The well-being or benefit of the individual ought to be promoted.
- The Principle of Non-maleficence. One ought to do no harm.
- The Principle of Justice. Equals ought to be considered equally.
- Non-therapeutic research. Experimental design does not benefit participants directly.
- Therapeutic research. Participants may obtain therapeutic benefit from taking part in the study.
- Consequentialism. There is one ultimate moral aim, that outcomes be as good as possible.
- Kant's Categorical Imperative. 'Act only on the maxim which you can at the same time will that it should become a universal law'.
- Informed consent. Voluntary agreement by an adequately informed, autonomous person, to investigation or treatment.

Access to health care: the QALY and its alternatives

'Health care systems, irrespective of how they are financed, present the paradox that to some observers they appear as a major component of social benefits, while to other observers they seem both excessively costly and limited in their effectiveness.' [1]

Learning outcomes

After reading this chapter, you should be able to:
* Identify macro- and micro-economic questions related to the allocation of resources within the National Health budget.
* Critically appraise the notion of 'finite' resource.
* List the criteria upon which access to treatment are currently based and discuss their morality.
* Critically discuss the moral arguments raised by the notional use of the QALY.
* Describe alternatives and solutions which may assist a more moral approach to resource allocation and treatment access.

14.1 INTRODUCTION

Advances in medical knowledge, skills and technology have made it possible to treat or prevent a number of diseases previously associated with a high mortality, resulting in a trend towards an increased proportion of elderly individuals within the population. Bury[2] has projected that there will be a two-thirds increase in the number of over 85 year olds in the UK between 1985 and the millennium. Concerns have been expressed that the development of measures, such as the QALY (quality adjusted life year), may limit their access to health care resources[3]. What is the basis for resource allocation and how could such a state of affairs arise?

With the inauguration of the welfare state in 1948, the philosophy of health care provision funded by taxation was based on meeting individual needs, arising from considerations of equity and justice. Currently in the UK, we spend about 6% of the gross national product on health care, one of the lowest figures for European countries (France 8.5%, Greece 3.9%). In comparison, the percentage expenditure on health care by Denmark, Germany and Sweden is 136, 163 and 229% above the UK figure. Reasons advanced for our low expenditure in comparison with other countries include a more efficient use of resources, with practitioners controlling access to expensive treatments and diagnostic procedure; raising revenue by taxation, and political fiscal control[1]. In determining the national health budget, the percentage of the GNP expenditure on health care requires justification against other vital items – defence, housing and education. Commenting on the discrepancy between need and the finite nature of resources for health care, Owen stated:

> '... if the need is not infinite, it is certainly so large relative to the resources which society is able to provide now and in the foreseeable future, that we can never hope to meet it completely'.[5]

14.2 MACRO- AND MICRO-ECONOMIC ISSUES

Macroeconomic decisions are predominantly the province of politicians, designed to provide answers to questions such as how much of the GNP should be spent on the health budget? How should this be partitioned between community and institutional settings? To what treatments should it be distributed? Commenting on the finite nature of resources and the political control of macroeconomic issues, Rawles[6] has stated that it is not obvious why the health budget (% GNP) is fixed at a level for which no strong electoral mandate exists. Increasing total resources to the NHS could simplify decisions on the partition of money. Rawles also questions the true 'finite' nature of resources, since epidemiological surveys can now confirm and predict with accuracy statistics for the incidence of disease, its associated morbidity and mortality, together with the nature and costs of treatment. Furthermore, Lamb[7] has suggested that, inflation apart, the NHS requires only about a 2 % increase in funding to keep pace with demographic and technological changes, a figure which is far from infinite.

In the decisions concerned with partition of the health care budget amongst different types of treatments, priorities must be considered in relation to resources. Exactly who makes these decisions? Recent NHS changes have resulted in the transfer of decision making on some of these crucial issues to managers and accountants. Black has emphasised how essential interpretation of clinical issues is to informed decision making and questions the involvement of individuals without the appropriate skills or professional judgement. Stressing the personal and human skills required for decision making Black comments that:

> '... procedures and attitudes which may be appropriate for managing a chain store are unlikely to be appropriate in a health service'.[1]

Where resources are limited and the delivery of high-quality, cost-effective care is an important consideration, the issue of measurement of treatment outcomes arises. Considerations of beneficence and non-maleficence support requirements to know which treatments benefit patients most. What may constitute favourable outcomes can be interpreted in different ways – duration of survival, quality of life, diminished tumour growth, chemotherapy relatively free from side-effects and capacity for employment, are examples of measures which have been used. To know how treatments compare in terms of benefit is useful; however, outcome measures can also be used to prioritise treatments for resource allocation, and in the case of the measure known as the QALY, to select individuals for treatment who are most likely to benefit from it, which raises serious moral questions (see 6.2.). At the level of microeconomics, who will get the treatment and what criteria (if any) should be applied to individuals, are emotive, controversial questions. Mooney[8] has emphasised the need to debate these carefully and consider alternatives dispassionately, since rhetoric and 'shroud waving' are unlikely to produce an equitable, just allocation of resources. The following case examples illustrate the moral dilemmas raised by having to choose between individuals.

Case study 1

An elderly man aged 70 years is admitted to hospital with a history of progressively deteriorating chronic renal failure. Renal function tests confirm that he has reached end-stage renal failure for which dialysis is a life-saving intervention. Only one bed is available on the renal dialysis unit; his case for treatments is considered alongside that of a young mother with two school-aged children. He is not selected for treatment.

Case study 2

A new form of chemotherapy is developed for lung cancer which is highly effective and relatively safe from side-effects. Stratified, randomised, clinical trials show conclusively that it is just as effective in the 'young elderly' between 65–70 years of age as in a group over 85 years of age. An oncology clinic based at a local district general hospital has limited supplies of this drug, which is expensive. More patients in the younger age group are selected for chemotherapy.

Such cases raise serious questions in relation to discrimination against the elderly, and the violation of ethical principles of justice as fairness, beneficence, non-maleficence and respect for autonomy (see 1.5). In the cases cited above, age *per se* and age linked to judgements about the value of an individual's life appear to have informed decision making. What criteria are currently used to determine access to treatment at the individual level, and how do these compare with those encapsulated in the QALY?

14.3 CURRENT CRITERIA INFORMING CHOICE

Stoll[9] has reviewed some of the criteria used to inform decision making when selecting individuals for cancer treatment in the UK. These criteria include two major categories: tumour-based assessments and value judgements based on indirect assessments. The former can include tumour size, and/or spread linked to the presence of life-threatening symptoms, the degree of effectiveness which treatment options could have on these. Stoll comments that due to the uncertainties inherent in treatment, risks exist that medical paternalism or prejudice may bias the information given to patients concerning alternatives to therapy. Of the indirect assessments, general medical status, quality of life, age and usefulness to the community may be used, all of which can be unsatisfactory. Quality of life measurements may be limited in scope and fail to consider individual patient's views; functional status may provide a more useful criteria than chronological age; the use of social class, economic and employment status, raise issues of social justice in that those who are better educated could be perceived to be of more use to the community and could be advantaged.

Stoll[9] has noted that the variety of value judgements used in conjunction with diverse clinical assessments can lead to inconsistencies in the selection of individuals for treatment between medical practitioners. Again, inequity and considerations of justice as fairness are raised. Possible approaches to removing such inequities could include the following:

- Development of standardised guidelines for the management of cancer treatment and other life-threatening illnesses.
- Codes of practice developed by independent multidisciplinary committees which identify criteria for resource allocation.
- Debate, consultation and approval by society of criteria used in resource allocation.

14.4 PROPOSED INSTRUMENTS; THE QALY REVISITED

The development of the QALY was an attempt by economists to devise a method of measuring life-enhancing and extending aspects of treatment[10]. Its basis was founded in assigning certain medical treatments a QALY value which corresponded to the number of QALYs a patient could experience with treatment minus the number of QALYs if left untreated. It was then possible to calculate the cost of each QALY gained in these calculations (see 6.2.3).

A year of healthy life expectancy was taken to be worth 1.0, and a year of unhealthy life expectancy to be less than 1.0, its value diminishing as quality of life decreased in the unhealthy.

Examples of QALY values of different treatments included the following:
- Heart transplants: 4.5 QALYs at £5,000.
- Total hip replacement: 4.0 QALYs at £700 per QALY.
- Home-renal dialysis: 6.0 QALYs at £14,000 per QALY[10].

From an economic perspective, beneficial, cost-effective, high-priority health care activities can be viewed as those generating the most QALYs at the lowest cost, that is, on the basis of the figures cited above, total hip replacement. The concept of the QALY had its potential uses and has provided a controversial source of debate in the literature on medical economics and ethics for almost a decade. What are the moral arguments against its use? Are there any benefits to be gained? What are the alternatives to the QALY?

Benefits of the QALY

Economists, while accepting that there may be flaws in QALY design, stress the benefits of contemplating their use[8]. Health care practitioners also concede that they can be useful in concentrating attention on the moral issues raised. Therefore, perceived benefits are:
- to place an emphasis on resource limitation;

- to stress that measuring health care outputs is important;
- to draw attention to the fact that interpersonal comparisons of utility can be made in decision making;
- to focus attention on the potential for violation of principles of justice in decision making.

Mooney[8] views the goal as developing better QALYs to assist decision making, but also suggests that QALYs are not the sole output to be considered in evaluating health care. Other important utilities for consideration beyond the QALY relate to the provision of information and empowerment in decision making by patients. How can these outputs be measured?

Objectives to the QALY

Objectives can be considered on grounds of both morality and the assumptions and flaws inherent in QALY construction.

ASSUMPTIONS

Health is viewed/equated as a state of 'good' life expectancy, freedom from pain, disability, and employment. This can be challenged on the basis that it is quality not solely quantity of life that is crucial. Health means different things to different individuals and is a complex construct. Disabled individuals do not necessarily view themselves as less healthy.

FLAWS

The quality of life measures used in the development of the QALY focused on criteria such as mobility, reduced pain, length of life and employment[12]. These are very limited aspects of the social, psychological, physical, spiritual and other dimensions of life which can be used in such assessments, which also need to consider individual weightings to enhance reliable interpretation.

MORAL ARGUMENTS

- QALYs are based on consequentialist calculations of benefit in selectively funding treatments; some individuals/groups in society will therefore lose out on health care.
- The violation of autonomy in decision making and the potential for selecting only those who are younger, healthier and most able to maximise benefits of treatment is unjust(see Chapter 6).
- Basing health care delivery and resource allocation on such consequentialist principles would have a negative impact on caring relationships between health professionals and the recipients of care.
- Health professionals are committed by virtue of professional ethical codes to respect autonomy and act beneficently and non-maleficently to recipients of care. Use of the QALY could create insoluble moral friction where needy individuals do not receive care.
- The use of QALYs imposes the subjective values of others on an individual's life plan, which is set aside. This is a morally objectionable violation of autonomy [14].
- QALYs focus on quality and length of life, omitting to consider its value and uniqueness in an individual[15].
- Use of QALYs could lead to a rapid decline down the slippery slope, to a point

where access to treatment is based on punitive or retributive principles which also violate autonomy. For example, restricting access to renal dialysis machines by vagrants or drug addicts, charging hospital costs to smokers with lung cancer[16].

14.5 ALTERNATIVES?

Harris[15] has suggested that the only equitable approach to select individuals for treatment where resources are limited is to randomise access. Is this a practical solution? Seedhouse[16] has commented that this could offend some views that exceptionally special circumstances must operate if one person is to be treated rather than another.

14.6 SOCIETY MUST DECIDE?

Chapter 6 (in the analysis of the interpretation of justice proposed by Rawls) suggested that society should determine principles of justice as fairness from behind a veil of 'ignorance', that is, a position removed from bias.

In resolving the ethical problems created by rationing scarce medical resources, it has been argued that society must approve the basis for identifying priorities, since they are society's resources which are used in health care. It must not be assumed that society has delegated this task to health care professionals or economists[8, 9]. How are societies views to be obtained? Lewis and Cherney[17] suggested that surveys of public opinion by remote questioning should provide a guide to prioritisation in medical care. These authors conducted such a survey of randomly selected members of the public in Cardiff. Participants were asked how they would choose between individuals of different ages suffering from the same life-threatening diseases. The finding that the majority of the sample selected younger in preference to older persons was concluded to support the notion that society operates a utilitarian approach to access scarce medical resources. However, the results also demonstrated that choices were less certain where age differences were closer. A similar experiment carried out in Oregon, USA, surveyed public opinion on prioritisation of treatments which they would support in terms of financial resources. Preventative health care programmes were favoured in comparison with high-technology treatments, and antenatal support of mothers was preferred in comparison with the intensive (and costly) support of premature babies whose prognosis was poor.

How relevant are these findings? Whitaker[18] suggested that they are irrelevant due to the social distancing of respondents, and bear no relation to that of decision making in a situation where, for example, a family member would be the recipient of such a decision. In such a situation it is argued, respondents would answer differently. Almond[19] concluded that it would have been more appropriate if respondents had asked themselves prior to choosing, 'Is what I propose to say useful or helpful to those confronting the problem personally?' A further point here is what would constitute useful research to assist decision making? Almond emphasised that we need to identify what principles people do use in considering rights of access to treatment and the elucidation of such principles, together with their interaction, may identify practical solutions. Analysis of practical cases could also generate broad principles. A final point rebutting the view that society would operate a utilitarian approach to resource allocation has been made by Whitaker[18] in relation to the considerable funding of charitable research, institutional and community care made possible by society's donations. This suggests that considerations which are exclusively utilitarian in nature do not operate amongst members of society.

14.7 CONCLUSIONS

Exceptionally difficult moral decisions must be made in the current environment of health care provision. Positive action in relation to the following proposals may clarify the moral issues and provide a starting point for the resolution of inequality.

- Society must be consulted and debate the criteria upon which resource allocations are to be made.
- Standardised guidelines should be developed for the management of life-threatening diseases.
- Codes of practice developed by multidisciplinary committees, including lay representatives, should identify criteria for resource allocation and treatment access.
- Current funding should be reviewed and audit procedures implemented to identify cost savings.
- Information obtained from reliable epidemiological data should be utilised to predict resource requirements for treatment in the NHS and to clarify formulation of a finite health budget.
- Above all, health care practitioners, economists and managers must be educated to reason morally. This is a vital prerequisite for the delivery of high-quality health care in a just society.

LEARNING EXERCISES

1. Discuss the funding basis of the NHS. Explain how inequalities can arise in access to care.
2. Discuss the morality of using tumour-based assessments and value judgements in selecting patients for cancer treatment.
3. Critically appraise the benefits, assumptions and moral objections inherent in the use of the QALY.
4. 'Ethics the heart of health care?' Discuss in relation to resource allocation and treatment access.
5. Discuss the implications for professional, caring relationships in relation to the proposed use of the QALY.

REFERENCES

1. Black, D. (1991). 'Paying for health'. *Journal of Medical Ethics*, **17**:117–23.
2. Bury, M. (1988). Arguments about ageing; long life and its consequences. In N. Neils and Freer (eds) *The Ageing Population*. Macmillan, London, UK.
3. Jeffreys, M. (1993). 'Geriatric medicine; some issues concerned with its development'. In A. Crabb (Ed.) *Choices and Decisions in Health Care*. John Wiley, Chichester, UK.
4. Maynard, A. (1988). 'Financing healthcare within the NHS?' *Cardiology Management*, **1**: 29–31.
5. Owen, D. (1976). *In Sickness and in Health; The Politics of Medicine*. Quartet Books, London, UK.
6. Rawles, J. (1989). 'Castigating QALYs.' *Journal of Medical Ethics*, **15**: 143–7.
7. Lamb, D. (1990). 'A plea for a touch of realism'. *Journal of Medical Ethics*, **16**:134–5.

8. Mooney, G. (1989). 'QALYS: are they enough? A health economists perspective'. *Journal of Medical Ethics*, **15**: 148–52.
9. Stoll, B.A. (1990). 'Choosing between cancer patients'. *Journal of Medical Ethics*, **16**: 71–4.
10. Williams, A. (1985). 'Economics of coronary artery by pass grafting'. *British Medical Journal*, **291**:326–9.
11. Seedhouse, D. (1986). *Ethics, The Heart of Health Care*. John Wiley, Chichester.
12. Rosser, R. and Kind, P. (1978). 'A scale of valuation of states of illness, is there a consensus?' *International Journal of Epidemiology*, **7**: 347–57.
13. Goodinson, S.M. and Singleton, J. (1989). 'Quality of life: a critical review of current concepts, measures and their clinical implications'. *International Journal of Nursing Studies*, **26**(4): 327–41.
14. Brown, J., Kitson, A.L. and McKnight, T. (1992). *Challenges in Caring: Explanation in Nursing and Ethics*. Chapman & Hall, London.
15. Harris, J. (1985). *The Value of Life*. Routledge & Kegan Paul, London.
16. Lockwood, M. (1988) *Quality of Life and Resource Allocation*. Proceedings, University of York Conference on Moral Philosophy in Health Care, September 1988.
17. Lewis, P.A. and Cherney, M. (1989) 'Which of two individuals do you treat when their ages are different and you can't treat them both?' *Journal of Medical Ethics*, **15**: 28–32.
18. Whitaker, P. (1990) 'Resource allocation – a plea for a touch of realism'. *Journal of Medical Ethics*, **16**:129–31.
19. Almond, B. (1988) 'Philosophy, medicine and its technologies'. *Journal of Medical Ethics*, **14**:173–8.

Key points

- Quality Adjusted Life Year (QALY). A measure of life extending and enhancing aspects of treatment for a given medical condition.
- The Prinicple of Justice. Equals ought to be considered equally.
- The Principle of Autonomy. In certain areas an individual has a right to be self-governing.
- The Principle of Beneficence. The well-being or benefit of the individual ought to be promoted.
- The Principle of Non-maleficence. One ought to do no harm.
- Consequentialism. There is one ultimate moral aim, that outcomes be as good as possible.

CHAPTER 15

Professional codes of conduct, accountability and advocacy

'Professional morality requires something of its members which general morality would not expect of lay persons.' [1]

Learning outcomes

After reading this chapter, you should be able to:
- Discuss the function of professional codes of conduct.
- Identify the strengths and limitations of professional codes.
- Clinically appraise the relationships of codes to moral principles.
- Discuss the ethical and professional rationales for advocacy.
- Describe limitations and identify alternatives for professional advocacy roles.

15.1 INTRODUCTION

One of the time-honoured definitions of a health profession is that it utilises a research-based body of knowledge vital to human welfare and need. Another is that its members subscribe to a code of conduct which provides an ethical framework stating how professionals should behave to recipients of care, each other and society (see 1.4). Essentially, professional codes function to provide:
- Guidelines for self-regulation in the maintenance of high standards.
- Confidence, reassurance and support to society concerning the ideals underpinning conduct and practice.
- A framework for decision making which enshrines contemporary views of professional morality.

Rumbold [2] makes the point that it is important to discriminate between a code of ethics and a code of conduct. The former incorporates statements affirming professional belief and commitment in high standards of conduct. The latter is:

'... a code of guidance regarding appropriate conduct for a specific group of people carrying out specific actions'.[3, 4]

A code of conduct usually incorporates general statements related to the ethical principles underpinning both professional duties and patients' rights on issues such as informed consent, confidentiality and privacy. The interpretation of these statements is intended to guide professional conduct and moral obligations within caring relationships of trust, worth and dignity.

15.2 TEMPORAL CHANGES

In relation to codes of practice, Black has commented that 'medical ethics are relative and not absolute for all time'[5]. A historical review of professional codes demonstrates how they have reflected the influence of contemporary society together with perceptions of professional issues and morality. For example, the ICN Code of Ethics in 1965 suggested that nurses 'carried out the physician's orders'; by 1973 the revised codes stressed the egalitarianism of the profession, the need to exercise judgement and reflect critically upon practice. In contrast, declarations of the World Medical Association have emphasised that doctors held 'the most respect for human life from the time of conception'[6, 7]. From 1983 the declaration accepted that attitudes to the life of the unborn child were 'a matter of individual conviction and conscience which must be respected'[8].

15.3 SCOPE, ACCOUNTABILITY, LIMITATIONS

Muyskens[9] emphasised that professional codes set the boundaries and outline the ideals for practice. They are not intended to provide comprehensive answers to all the situations a professional will encounter in the performance of practice or attempt to make individual decisions for them. Features identified as necessary in such codes are comprehension, brevity and acceptability/generalisability in relation to assent of the profession, together with sufficient flexibility to allow freedom and respect for the autonomy of the professional in decision making. The UKCC[10] view of one principle purpose of the professional code is to enable members to exercise accountability, the process of making judgements about actions which have outcomes calculated to benefit the individual (see Appendix 2). From a legal perspective, accountability can be defined as the extent to which the health professional can be held in law, to account for their actions[11]. Specific areas of accountability relate to the general public, the profession, recipients of care and the employer, in all of which practitioners can be held liable for any negligent action

The UKCC Code of Conduct for Nurses, Midwives and Health Visitors[10] supplementary advisory document on exercising accountability, lays a particular emphasis on accountability in the areas of: environments of care; consent and truth; advocacy, collaboration and co-operation in care; and conscientious objection. How do these implicitly relate to ethical principles?

Environments of care

'Nurses, midwives and health visitors must act to serve the interest of society and

above all to safeguard the interests of individuals in their care'.[10]

Where environments are unsuitable or poorly resourced placing recipients of care, staff and standards of practice at risk, they should make representations to their immediate professional manager. These interventions are justified by the principles of beneficence and non-maleficence, wherein the professional actions are for the benefit or well-being of the individual and are intended to remove harm (see 5.1, 5.2). Considerations of justice also apply here since resources may not have been distributed in fairness, according to the needs of recipients of care or staff (see 6.1).

Consent and truth

Accountability here relates to treatments or procedures for which informed consent should be obtained from the individual, that is, after adequate information and honest explanation have been given, following which understanding has been ascertained (see 12.2). Recognition is also given to truth telling in relation to the condition of individuals and the duty to provide information which is in their interest (see page 00). Both facets of accountability referred to can be justified on moral grounds by the principle of respect for autonomy and the need to treat recipients of care as ends in themselves (see 4.1, 4.2.1, 4.2.2.) Again, the principles of beneficence and non-maleficence also apply (see 5.1, 5.2).

Objection to participation in care and treatment

Situations can arise in professional duties, where the practitioner chooses not to participate in a form or aspect of treatment on the grounds of conscience. Under the law, practitioners can exert this right solely in relation to the procedure of termination of pregnancy. The important ethical precept at issue here is respect for the autonomy of the practitioners in relation to views concerning the sanctity of life (see 4.2, 9.1, 9.1.2).

Occasionally, a practitioner may refuse to participate in the care of a patient suffering from a serious condition such as AIDS. Here, the UKCC's views are unequivocal: practitioners are expected to adopt a non-judgemental approach in the exercise of their caring role[10]. Observation of this tenet is justified on grounds of respect for the person, impartiality, justice as fairness, beneficence and non-maleficence (see 4.2, 5.1, 5.2).

Collaboration and co-operation in care

Clause 5 of the Code of Professional Conduct (see Appendix) underlines the vital importance of teamwork in a spirit of positive co-operation which will enhance the delivery of high-quality care. This is justified by the principle of respect for autonomy, which is essential for the survival of relationships which we have with other people (see 4.4). Respect for autonomy can be justified on deontological grounds (see 4.2.2) and also on the consequentialist basis that this will maximise benefits, in this case, in relation to the patient and team decision making (see 4.2.1, 16.1).

In general, criticism of professional codes of conduct is frequently directed at their perceived lack of specificity, the fact that conflict can arise in the observation of clauses (see 1.4) and that they do not provide a basis for moral decision making. Counter arguments to these points have been omitted above in the case of the UKCC. The suggestion has been made that to avoid accusations of paternalistic elitism, we should base regulation of the profession on a contract with the community rather than with a self-regulatory committee. Public participation in the development of professional codes could then take place.

Another important issue concerns the effectiveness of codes. Are codes violated because some health professionals are powerless to control practice in the power hierarchy in which they work? Ethical principles inherent in codes may conflict with authoritarian values in institutional power structures. These reasons are frequently advanced to explain why some health professionals cannot assume an advocacy role.

15.4 ADVOCACY

'In the exercise of professional accountability, the practitioner will accept a role as an advocate on behalf of his/her patients or clients'.[10]

Although strong emphasis is laid by the UKCC on the role of the nurse as the patients advocate, little guidance is offered in its interpretation for it asserts that each practitioner must determine exactly how this aspect of accountability is satisfied in his or her practice[10]. Could permitting individual interpretations of such statements lead to variable practice and inconsistency in standards of accountability? Since situations which require advocacy can give rise to enormous conflicts, as described in the case example below, this role requires careful moral deliberation.

The staff nurse example

A staff nurse on night duty at a geriatric long-stay hospital is responsible, with the help of one auxiliary nurse, for the care of 30 highly dependent individuals. Many are in persistent vegetative states, are confused or senile and require considerable attention. Due to staffing shortages not all the patients' needs can be met at an acceptable standard. The hospital managers are made aware of the problem but fail to employ more staff. The nurse complains to the UKCC and Health Service Commissions and a formal enquiry attracting adverse media coverage is held. The findings support the complaints made, the ward is closed and amid a great deal of unpleasant professional conflict the nurse loses her job.

What ethical questions have arisen for the nurse in this example? How can advocacy be interpreted here? The ethical principles which underpin such questions are beneficence, non-maleficence, justice and autonomy. (see 4.2.1, 5.2, 6.1). The nurse's actions are motivated by concern that beneficence and non-maleficence are violated. The best interests of the recipients of care are not being served and harm may result as a consequence of the inadequate quality of care engendered by low staffing levels. The treatment delivered is neither equitable nor fair; rights to safe care, dignity and respect for the person are being abused. An important aspect of the nursing role here is in acting as a representative for the individuals who in this case have diminished autonomy[12]. According to Brower an advocate is also one who 'defends, pleads the cause of, or changes systems on behalf of an individual or group'[13]. Inherent in this definition are activities that are aimed at a redistribution of power and resources. In the 'staff nurse example', the nurse is also acting as an advocate for the individual' rights in defending their needs for adequately resourced care.

In a different context, advocacy can also encompass:

> '... *informing the patient of his/her rights in a particular situation; ensuring he/she has all the necessary information to make an informed decision; supporting him/her in the decision taken; protecting and safeguarding the patient's interests.'*[14]

Here the individual's right to self-rule – autonomy – is positively emphasised, the role of the nurse being to support the them in making decisions in accordance with his/her values after critical reflection. These decisions might relate to treatment options, discontinuation of treatments, or requests to be told the truth about one's diagnosis (see 12.3). Since individuals' decisions may not coincide with the views of other health care professionals, this may place the nurse in a position of professional conflict. Advocacy in the context of individuals' rights can also mean informing them of those contained in the Patients' Charter[15], since some may be unaware of this.

Justifications and objections

Carpenter[16] has identified five categories of patients who may require an advocate. These include those who are handicapped, immature, acutely ill, inhibited from requesting information and those with limited knowledge. Are nurses ideally placed to fulfil an advocacy role for these categories of patients?

A number of questions have arisen in relation to the assumption of an advocacy role for nurses. Arguably, this role is supported by ethical principles inherent in the professional code of conduct and the nature of the therapeutic relationship, which is one of trust and can involve considerable day-to-day contact. In order to function effectively in an advocacy role it is necessary to be non-judgmental, impartial and place the individual's interests above the professional's own; emotional neutrality should be adopted towards the recipient of care[17]. In addition, introspection about one's own motivation, knowledge and skills linked to self-knowledge of one's own value system is essential.

Problems can arise where the therapeutic relationship is perceived to be unequal. The relationship can be one of dependence and the recipient of care may feel loss of personal control, by virtue of his/her medical condition and its impact on life plans. Part of the nursing role can involve promotion or acceptance of medical treatments which introduce elements of vulnerability to coercion and persuasion[19]. In this context, advocacy could lead to paternalism on the part of the nurse[20]. Assumption of the advocacy role could also lead to increased dependency by individuals, when self-advocacy should be the ultimate goal in encouraging a person to attain independence[21]. Clearly, some individuals cannot attain this and will never be self-advocates.

There are a number of other concerns about assumption of the advocacy role which include the following. Nurses are not legally trained to plead and defend the cause of another. Alternative models of advocacy have been proposed in which specially trained, independent legal counsellors fulfil this role, entirely free of institutional bias. A critical point here is that the recipient of care should be allowed to exercise free will in choosing an advocate to represent his/her interests, that is, advocates are mandated[20].

In addition, the bureaucratic, hierarchical institutional settings in which nurses practise, linked to their concerns about employment, may act as a disincentive to publicise bad practice. Porter has commented that:

> '... nurses may not be capable of conceding their vested interests, or challenging
> the vested interests of their colleagues. Schism and conflict can arise in
> professional relationships between nurses and other health care professionals, who
> may also feel they have a legitimate advocacy role for those in their care.'[21]

15.5 RIGHTS

As discussed above, advocacy can encompass:

> '... informing the patient of his/her rights in a particular situation; ensuring
> he/she has all the necessary information to make an informed decision, protecting
> and safeguarding the patients interest'.[14]

Such definitions raise a number of issues for the practitioner. Is the recipient of care autonomous, rational, competent and how has this been determined? What reasonable information should be given to enable a decision to be made? Has the individual indicating their wishes to be involved in decision making? If the person is not competent what consultation process is necessary to enable a decision to be made and to safeguard the individual's interests? A crucial question concerns also the issue of rights: what rights do the recipients of health care actually possess?

In general, 'rights' are considered to be features of a civilised society. Childress[22] suggests that the principle of respect for autonomy (see 4.2) generates several right, or 'justified claims against others'. The concept of the assertion of claims suggests that a mechanism must exist whereby claims are recognised. In turn, these may require other persons to act or refrain from acting and, in addition, place certain obligations upon them. A distinction can be made between moral rights which can be justified by ethical principles, and legal rights justified by legal principles established by Acts of Parliament.

Moral rights are enshrined in respect for the autonomy of rational agents (Kant see 4.2.2), liberty and freedom (Mill, see 4.2.1) and concepts of 'life, liberty and estate' proposed by Locke in the seventeenth century[23]. Moral rights can arise from 'general, collective, morally intuitive judgements', for example, in relation to slavery or killing people[24]. However, such rights can be interpreted in different ways, for example, rights of life of a fetus can be accepted or rejected on the basis of arguments concerned with personhood (see 10.3). The moral basis for rights in relation to health care are based on the Principles of Justice, Autonomy, Beneficence and Non-maleficence and are explored in detail in Chapters 4–6. Furthermore, codes of professional conduct place moral obligations upon health care professionals in relation to those in their care.

Distinct from moral rights are legal rights, established or disestablished by Parliamentary Act. For many, these are viewed as the only rights worth having, since they offer the prospect of legal enforcement by a claimant. Although the UK is a signatory to the European Convention of Human Rights, our legal system does not directly recognise or enforce its clauses, and neither has the UK established its own

'Bill of Rights'. Examples of some key rights are summarised in **Table 15.1**; not included here are rights in relation to privacy, investigation of complaints and rights of citizens detained under the Mental Health Act 1983. Not all legal rights are absolutely enforceable and, in many, the responsibility lies with the individual to offer incontrovertible proof of negligence or trespass to be successful in prosecuting a claim. Use of the Bolam Test (12.2.1) and the recognition of therapeutic privilege by the courts can limit the extent to which claimants can be prosecuted.

The concept of rights in relation to health care is a relatively new. Invested awareness of the need for enforceable rights has been created by a number of factors:

- The rise of consumerism linked to the view of active participation in health care decision making by its recipients (see Chapter 17).
- Formation of community Health Councils which have solicited consumer views about the health service and the establishment of a Health Service Ombudsman to investigate complaints.
- Perceived needs for protection against paternalistic infringement of the autonomy of competent individuals by health professionals.
- Empowerment of those whose autonomy may be constrained.
- Increased public awareness through the establishment of Acts, such as the Mental Health Act 1983, which gives careful consideration to the autonomy of detained individuals in relation to treatment.
- Advances in medical science have raised expectations of health care; the development of technologies which can artificially extend life has raised issues about rights to die and to refuse treatment.
- Concerns raised by a rise in iatrogenic disease associated with medical treatments[25].

In 1992, the inception of the Patient's Charter[15] suggested that consumers of health care possessed certain rights in relation to treatment. Have these a legal status in terms of enforceability? Currently, health care consumers do not possess contractual rights, purchasing power or the power to enforce statutory duties[26]. Furthermore, consumer law does not apply to health care, where the Bolam Test can be used to decide what is reasonable in terms of claimant's rights, for example, in relation to negligence (see Table 15.1). However, positive benefits of the Patient's Charter could be derived from its use in standard settings as part of quality assurance schemes, where health care outcomes are carefully monitored.

In conclusion, the need for protection of autonomy and consumer rights in clinical decision making is paramount, especially for vulnerable groups. Powerful arguments exist to suggest an independent advocacy system may offer the most acceptable method of provision.

LEARNING EXERCISES

1. Are professional codes of conduct useful in ethical decision making?
2. Define 'accountability'. What are its professional and ethical implications?
3. Critically discuss the role of the nurse in relation to advocacy.
4. Discuss with strong justification the moral principles that you would include in a professional code of conduct.
5. Critically discuss the suggestion that professional bodies should not be self-regulatory.

Table 15.1 Examples of key legal rights

Right	Legal basis	Comment
1. Rights to health care and medical assistance	Statutory duties of the Secretary of State enshrined in the NHS Acts of 1948 and 1977	In general, not enforceable except where claims of negligence may be brought due to (1) failure of a GP to attend a patient who suffers harm, (2) failure of ambulance services to arrive leading to harm
2. Rights to receive reasonable care	Proof of negligence requires compensation (Law of Tort)	Negligence is not easy to establish. The Bolam Test (see Chapter 12) applies in relation to standards of care
3. Rights to consent to treatment and to refuse treatment	Trespass to the person	Voluntary, informed consent by an autonomous individual is a defence to an action for trespass, as are common law powers to act out of necessity and those incorporated in the Mental Health Act 1983
	Negligence	Information giving standards assessed using the Bolam Test; courts recognise medical therapeutic privilege
4. Rights of access to health records	Data Protection Act 1984; Access to Medical Reports Act 1988; Access to Health Records Act 1990	Access rights incorporate inspection of records, making copies, explanation of medical terms used
		Access can be denied if information is likely to cause harm or involves the identification of other individuals who have not given consent to disclosure
		Therapeutic privilege applied to the acts
5. Confidentiality	Duty of care Employment contracts (implied duties) Duties based on equity	Confidentiality is incorporated in professional codes of conduct; exceptions to the confidentiality of information are summarised in Chapter 12

REFERENCES

1. Brown, J., Kitson, A.L. and McKnight, T. (1992). *Challenges in Caring*. Chapman & Hall, London.
2. Rumbold, G. (1993). *Ethics in Nursing Practice* (2nd edn). Bailliere Tindall, London.
3. Benjamin, M. and Curtis, J. (1992). *Ethics in Nursing* (3rd edn). Oxford University Press, Oxford.
4. Burnard, P. and Chapman, C. (1988). *Professional and Ethical Issues in Nursing*. J. Wiley, Chichester, UK.
5. Black, D. (1984) 'Iconoclastic ethics'. *Journal of Medical Ethics*, **10**: 179–82.
6. International Council of Nurses (1965, 1977) *Code for Nurses*. ICN, Geneva.
7. Declaration of Geneva (1965) World Medical Association, WMA Publications.
8. Declaration of Oslo (1983) World Medical Association, WMA Publications.
9. Muyskens, J.L. (1982). *Moral Problems in Nursing*. Rowman, Littlefield, UK.
10. UKCC (1992). *Professional Code of Conduct for Nurses, Midwives and Health Visitors*. UKCC, London.
11. Dimond, B. (1990). *Legal Aspects of Nursing*. Prentice Hall, London.
12. Abrams, N. (1978). 'A contrary view of the nurse as patient advocate'. *Nursing Forum*; XVII: **3**: 258–67.
13. Brower, H.T. (1982). 'Advocacy: what it is'. *Journal of Gerontological Nursing*, **8**(3):141–3.
14. Clark, J. (1982). 'Nursing matters: patient advocacy'. *Times Health Supplement*, 9 February.
15. Department of Health (1992) *The Patient's Charter: A Summary*. HMSO, London.
16. Carpenter, D. (1992). 'Advocacy'. Nursing Times, **88**:26–27.
17. Talcott Parsons (1976). In: *Hospitals, Paternalism and the Role of the Nurse*. Teachers College Press, New York.
18. Copp, L.A. (1986) 'The nurse as advocate for vulnerable persons'. *Journal of Advanced Nursing*, 11 May, 255–63.
19. Trandel–Korenchuk, D. and Trandel–Korenchuk, K. (1983). 'Nursing advocacy of patients' right: myth or reality. Parts 1 and 2'. *Nurse Practitioner*, **8**:53,55, 58–9 and **8**:4, 37, 40–2.
20. Allmark, P. (1992). The case against nurse advocacy. *British Journal of Nursing*, **2**(1), 33–6.
21. Porter, S. (1992). 'The poverty of professionalisation: a critical analysis of strategies for the occupational advance of nursing'. *Journal of Advanced Nursing*, **17**:720–6.
22. Childress, J. (1982). *Who Should Decide? Paternalism in Health Care*. Oxford University Press, Oxford, UK.
23. Carpenter, *op. cit.*
24. Gillon, R. (1986) *Philosophical Medical Ethics*. John Wiley, UK
25. Illich, I. (1975). *Medical Nemesis*. Pantheon Publications, New York.
26. Dimond, B. (1993). *Patients Rights, Responsbilities and the Nurse*. Quay Publishing, UK

Key points
- Accountability. The extent to which the health professional can be held in law to account for their actions.
- Advocacy. Defending the cause of an individual or group; informing patients of their rights.
- Informed consent. Voluntary agreement by an adequately informed, autonomous person, to investigation or treatment.
- The Principle of Beneficence. The well-being or benefit of the individual ought to be promoted.
- The Principle of Non-maleficence. One ought to do no harm.
- The Prnciple of Autonomy. In certain areas an individual has a right to be self-governing.
- The Sanctity of Life Principle. Life is of value and should not be destroyed.
- Consequentialism. There is one ultimate moral aim, that outcomes be as good as possible.
- Deontology. Certain prima facie duties such as truth-telling, non-maleficence, justice and beneficence are morally obligatory.
- Strong paternalism. Limiting or denying freedom of choice to a competent person capable of making an autonomous decision.
- The Principle of Justice. Equals ought to be considered equally.

CHAPTER 16

In the patient's interest?
Paternalism in health care

'No sauces ... no sweets ... no Attic pastry ... no Corinthian Girls!'

Plato, The Republic' *(a paternalistic edict on the pleasures of primary prevention)*

Learning outcomes

After reading this chapter, you should be able to:
- Define 'strong' and 'weak' paternalism and describe the situations in which it may affect decision making.
- Identify the concepts on which paternalism is based.
- Discuss the moral principles which are used to justify or refute paternalistic interventions.
- Identify moral principles which can take precedence in considering paternalistic interventions.
- Discuss specific arguments which can be used to justify or refute paternalism in truth telling, treatment decisions and primary prevention.

16.1 DEFINITIONS, BASIS FOR PATERNALISM

Trust and respect for the autonomy of individuals, it has been argued (see 12.1), are the vital foundation of the therapeutic relationship. A strong case has also been made for the principle of respect for autonomy and the importance of self-determination by rational, competent individuals in decisions affecting their medical treatment (see 4.2 and 4.2.2). Paternalism can be defined as:

> *'... a refusal to accept or to acquiesce in another person's wishes, choices or actions, for that persons benefit'.*[1]

On what grounds and in which situations could health professionals justify paternalistic interventions in the context of professional, caring relationships built on respect for autonomy? What is the origin of paternalism?

Paternalism is rooted in the biological model of a caring parent[2]. In the context of health care the professional who is acting paternalistically is engaging in benevolent actions which aim to maximise an individual's welfare; such actions involve making decisions on their behalf. Historically, paternalism has been associated with the individual being a passive recipient of health care, subsuming the quasi-child, 'sick-role', while that of the doctor has been viewed as that of active 'parent'.[3] From a sociological perspective, this assumption of care and control has been viewed negatively, as a legitimation of power in decision making by the health professional and health state[4]. A view of the doctor–patient therapeutic relationship which suggested that the need for paternalistic interventions should be adjusted across the autonomy–dependence continuum, and which described a move away from the historical, biomedical model was developed by Szasz and Hollander[5]. In this, doctor–patient interactions were classified as:

- Activity–passivity. Interaction minimal; patient passive; may be unable to make autonomous decisions. Doctor active; intervenes beneficently in acute illness, for example, unconscious individuals and life-threatening emergencies.
- Guidance–co-operation. Greater interaction occurs; individual acutely ill; temporarily intermittently incapacitated, seeks guidance from doctor. Doctor active in guiding or instructing during recovery.
- Mutual participation. Encountered in longer-term illness; individual exercises autonomy in decision making. Doctors interventions enabling; relationships equal, independent.

In recent years, the rise of consumerism has evoked a shift from the paternalistic, biomedical model of care to an autonomy model, which emphasises the rights of individuals in decision making and ensures that the preferences of consumers may not be over-ridden[6, 7]. While this has reinforced the mutual participation model of interactions between health professionals and consumers, it is important to bear in mind that some recipients of care may choose to waive their rights in decision making, and that there will always be others, for whom beneficent, paternalistic interventions are necessary and can be justified (see 16.5.3).

Paternalism can be viewed with varying degrees of dominance. 'Weak' paternalism occurs in situations where the health professional makes decisions which are in the interests of an individual whose autonomy is severely diminished and the paternalistic intervention holds the only hope of a positive outcome. For example, in life-threatening emergencies, such beneficent interventions by medical practitioners are morally acceptable and, indeed, obligatory. Lesser degrees of impaired autonomy can present some difficulties in assessment and the determination of a need for weak, paternalistic interventions. For example, in some forms of mental illness where florid delusions are present, individuals may retain rationality in relation to decision making about treatment and consent can be obtained (see 12.2.2).

In contrast, 'strong' paternalism involves either limiting or denying freedom of choice in health care decisions by a rational, competent individual who is capable of making an autonomous choice. The situations in which this can arise are varied, but can include limiting or removing autonomy in treatment selection (informed consent, see 12.2); withholding information and/or engaging in deception about a terminal diagnosis or poor prognosis (see 12.3.1); intervening in lifestyles or life plans as part of primary prevention in health education/promotion schemes.

16.2 MORAL JUSTIFICATIONS AND REFUTATIONS.

A number of moral principles can be brought into conflict in substantiating or refuting the need for paternalistic interventions.

16.2.1 Withholding 'bad news'

The rationale for withholding dire diagnostic or prognostic information from individuals suffering from a terminal illness is founded on the argument that to disclose this would cause misery and suffering. Appeals to the principles of beneficence and non-maleficence (see 4.3, 5.2, 5.5) are used to justify non-disclosure of information, which it is deemed is not in the individual's best interests to know and necessary to remove harm. A number of arguments can be advanced to counter this approach. Firstly, the principle of respect for the individual's autonomy has been violated. As argued in 4.2, this can be justified on both deontological and consequentialist grounds. Gillon[8] has emphasised the need for practitioners to utilise their therapeutic skills in discovering what individuals actually wish to know about their diagnosis and to act accordingly. In this, it is vital that consideration is given to the person's moral history, values and life plans[9]. Another important consideration here is that non-maleficent intentions in not revealing the truth may actually exacerbate suffering by consigning a patient to the uninformed limbo which can lead to anxiety and depression (see 12.3.1) [10, 11].

Furthermore, deception, once engaged, must be maintained, imposing further stress on carers. If deceit is discovered by an individual it can cause anger and suffering, undermining the foundation of the therapeutic relationship.

16.2.2 Treatment decisions

Paternalistic interventions in treatment decisions can appear in a number of forms. In extreme 'strong' cases, the medical practitioner decides what treatment is appropriate for the individual without consultation (informed consent, see 12.2). A more subtle approach may be, under the guise of choice, to provide the individual with information which is biased, and results in the selection of a treatment option which the medical practitioner considers to be in the individual's best interests.

Arguments which have been used to justify such paternalistic interventions are that, by virtue of the specialist knowledge and expertise acquired during training, medical practitioners are uniquely qualified to make such decisions and judge beneficently, what is the best treatment option. In contrast, recipients of care may have limited medical knowledge and therefore are assumed to be incapable of making truly informed decisions[12].

The justification for such interventions rests on the concept that the principle of beneficence takes precedence over considerations of respect for the patient's autonomy. The counter argument here is that the duty of beneficence should be constrained by respect for autonomy and that this requires the health professional to benefit and meet needs as defined by the patient's values; the pursuit of needs should be limited by the individual's wishes.[1] It has been argued that only the *informed* patient can *weigh* the benefits versus harms of treatment and the outcome may be different to that of the medical practitioner. If the individual's evaluation of benefits versus harms is coupled with the principle of beneficence (see 5.5) then this would also be in accordance with the principle of respect for autonomy. Additional considerations in the argument against paternalistic interventions include the point that medical judgement of responses to treatment can be fallible, and that doctors are not better able to judge what contributes to a person's quality of life in the context of treatment benefits; neither are they specially qualified to advise on moral decisions, where the individual's values are the prime consideration.[9]

The argument that individuals are not capable of understanding medical terminology, or of making informed decisions about treatment, is strongly refuted by the growing body of research-based knowledge accrued from patient education. This suggests that a number of effective methods can be used to inform individuals effectively about medical or nursing treatment and that this can benefit recovery in significant ways.[13, 14]

In recent years the developments related to individual rights, the rise of consumerism and concepts of active participation in treatment decisions would suggest that the pattern of paternalistic interventions in treatment decisions is changing. However, some research evidence suggests this is not entirely the case. Pinch and Spielman[15] surveyed the role of parents in ethical decision making in neonatal intensive care, by conducting interviews with families prior to the discharge of infants. Results of this survey suggested that parents adopted a passive role in decision making, which was acceptable for the majority, who conceded this to the professional expertise of medical staff. Although information sharing with parents had occurred in relation to treatment decisions, many could not remember this, possibly due to the anxiety-evoking situation. For this reason, information sharing should be reinforced at intervals and the extent to which parents wish to be involved should be re-explored. In contrast, Harrison[16] found that some parents strongly objected to non-involvement in decision making, and verbalised strong views about paternalistic infringements of autonomy and rights of parents/guardians to give informed consent. Pinch and Spielman[15] emphasised that it is imperative to identify parents who wish to be involved, and those who do not, at an early stage in treatment decisions. The outcomes of ethical decision making should then be monitored for families of both groups.

16.2.3 Primary prevention

Recent surveys have shown a decline in the incidence of coronary heart disease and its associated morbidity and mortality in the US. This has been attributed to the impact of programmes of primary prevention, which have focused on the modification of known 'lifestyle risk factors' such as smoking, inactivity and consumption of saturated dietary fat.[17, 18] How moral are such interventions? To what extent should behavioural modification be paternalistically endorsed or enforced? Childress[1] argued that programmes of primary prevention can infringe autonomy, respect for the person and liberty. In relation to the latter, Mill argued strongly against what can be construed as paternalistic interference and coercion in areas which were none of society's business.

> 'The only purpose for which power can be rightfully exercised over any member of a civilised community against his/her will is to prevent harm to others.' [19]

That is, respect for autonomy can be supported except where harm to others results. In relation to decisions which affect the quality of individuals' lives, it is vital that a person's moral values, life plan and evaluation of benefits versus harms are weighed.

> 'A person's life plan establishes the magnitudes of risk which he or she will accept for various ends.' [20]

A consideration of the individual's views, coupled with the principle of beneficence, would be in accord with respect for autonomy (see 5.5). On this basis, physicians and society should not interfere paternalistically with voluntary, self-regarding conduct. In relation to health education Clarke[21] emphasised that the role of the health educator must espose empowerment and respect for autonomy. Individuals should be assisted to clarify their own values and enabled to reach decisions relevant to their own situation and needs. Facilitation and empowerment of individuals hit at the heart of practice in health education. However, Childress[1] suggested that justified interventions could be made where risks of harm to others could result, for example, in relation to passive smoking.

LEARNING EXERCISES

1. Discuss the grounds on which weak paternalism could be justified.
2. Can paternalistic deception ever be justified in relation to truth telling?
3. Discuss the conflict between respect for autonomy and beneficence which arise in relation to paternalistic interventions. Which takes precedence?
4. Define paternalism and explain its conceptual basis.
5. Particular areas of moral behaviour are none of society's business. Discuss in relation to primary prevention.

REFERENCES

1. Childress, J.F. (1982) *Who Should Decide? Paternalism in Health Care*. Oxford University Press, Oxford.
2. Rothman, D.J. (1978) 'The state as parent: social policy in the progressive era'. In Gaylin, W. (ed.) *Doing Good: The Limits of Benevolence*. Pantheon Books, New York.
3. Parsons, T. (1951) *The Social System*. Free Press, New York.
4. Porter, S. (1992) 'The poverty of professionalisation: a critical analysis of strategies for the occupational advance of nursing'. *Journal of Advanced Nursing*, **17**:720–6.
5. Szasz, T. and Hollander, M. (1956) 'A contribution to the philosophy of medicine: 3 basic models of the doctor-patient relationship'. *Archives of Internal Medicine*, **97**:585–92.
6. Sutherland, H.J., Llewellyn–Thomas, H.A. and Lockwood, G.A. (1989) 'Cancer patients: their desire for information and participation in treatment decisions'. *Journal of the Royal Society of Medicine*, **82**:260–3.
7. Veatch, J.D. (1981). *A Theory of Medical Ethics*. Basic Books, New York
8. Gillon, R. (1986) *Philosophical Medical Ethics*. John Wiley, Chichester, UK.
9. Veatch, R.M. *op. cit.*
10. Dunbar, S. (1990) 'An obstructed death and medical ethics'. *Journal of Medical Ethics*, **16**: 83–7.

11. Higgs, R. (1990) 'An obstructed death and medical ethics'. *Journal of Medical Ethics*, **16**:90–2.
12. Gadow, S. (1989) 'An ethical case for patient self-determination'. *Seminars in Oncology Nursing*, **5**(2):99–101.
13. Wilson-Barnett, J., Fordham, M. (1982) *Recovery From Illness.* John Wiley, Chichester, UK.
14. Redman, B.K. (1980) *The Process of Patient Teaching in Nursing.* CV Mosby.
15 Pinch, W.J. and Spielman, M.L. (1990) 'The parent's perspective; ethical decision making in neonatal intensive care'. *Journal of Advanced Nursing*, **15**, 712–19.
16. Harrison, S. (1986) 'Neonatal intensive care: parent's role in ethical decision making'. *Birth*, **13**(3):165–75.
17. Morris (1977) 'Diet and heart.' *British Medical Journal*, **ii**,1307–14.
18. Dolecek, T.A. (1992) 'Current perspectives: cardiovascular nutrition education'. *Patient Education and Counselling*, **19**(1):3–4.
19. Mill, J.S. (1976) *On Liberty.* Himmelfarb, G. (ed). Penguin Books, London.
20. Clarke, J.B. (1993) 'Ethical issues in health education'. *British Journal of Nursing*, **2**(10): 533–8.

FURTHER READING

Ingelfinger, F. (1980) 'Arrogance'. *New England Journal of Medicine*, **303**:1507–11.
Parsons, T. (1976) Hospitals, *Paternalism and The Role of the Nurse.* Teachers College Press, New York.

Key points
- Strong paternalism. Limiting or denying freedom of choice to a competent person capable of making an autonomous decision.
- The Principle of Autonomy. In certain areas an individual has a right to be self-governing.
- Weak paternalism. Decisions are made by a health professional which are in the best interests of an individual who has diminished autonomy.
- The Principle of Beneficence. The well-being or benefit of the individual ought to be promoted.
- The Principle of Non-maleficence. One ought to do no harm.
- Consequentialism. There is one ultimate moral aim, that outcomes be as good as possible.
- Deontology. Certain prima facie duties such as truth-telling, non-maleficence, justice and beneficence are morally obligatory.

CHAPTER 7

Ethical decision making: professional and consumer perspectives

'If my mind could gain a foothold, I would not write essays, I would make decisions, but it is always in apprenticeship and on trial.'[1]

Learning outcomes

After reading this chapter, you should be able to:
* Define the scope and purpose of ethical decision making.
* Identify the ethical principles inherent in clinical decision making.
* Describe possible decision-making frameworks.
* Discuss the factors that can influence ethical decisions.
* Identify how effective team ethical decision making can improve patient care.

17.1 INTRODUCTION

Since health care is a moral endeavour, no health care professional can disclaim their involvement in ethical decision making. An apprenticeship in identifying and justifying the highest moral interventions possible in the diverse and challenging situations which can arise in health practice is a searching, illuminating and rewarding process. In essence, the intention throughout this entire text has been to present the reader with a range of moral problems which commonly arise in health care practice and to provide a firm foothold in considering the ethical principles which form the foundation for analysis and decision making. In this final chapter, further issues relevant to decision making are considered from the perspectives of the health care professional and consumer in the wider context of health care delivery. These include the scope of decision making; process principles, frameworks for moral deliberation and factors affecting decision making, including the notion of consumer rights.

17.2 DEFINITIONS, SCOPE AND PURPOSE OF DECISION MAKING

Griepp defines decision making as:

> '... a collaborative process based on sound information, within the realities of the client's works, where problems and conflicts are defined and delineated, and resolution is guided by ethical principles which respect the individual as an end in and of himself'.[2]

Implicit in this definition is the concept of partnership between the health care professional and client with respect for the client's autonomy guiding the decision-making process. In contrast, Seedhouse and Lovett[3] view the process of decision making as one of balancing theories against facts, precedents and opinions and consider stages in the process to be essentially the same for the doctor and recipient of care. For the former, clinical judgement and experience are seen to be crucial. Such are the definitions and purposes which guide health care delivery, the factors which underpin clinical judgement and the nature of professional relationships.

Central tenets of health care work are to respect and create patient or client autonomy, to minimise harm, to do positive good and to engage in interactions which produce the most beneficial outcomes for individuals or groups. Moral deliberation should then permeate all aspects of health care practice, not just life and death dilemmas but the mundane, everyday routines which may go unexamined. Levine emphasised that professional ethical behaviour is not:

> '... a display of moral rectitude in time of crises, but a day-by-day expression of one's commitment to other persons, and they ways in which human beings relate to one another in their daily interactions'.[4]

If health care professionals are to participate in the enabling, enhancing and empowering interventions which will preserve patient or client autonomy, a number of factors must inform approaches to decision making. These include a sound understanding of ethical principles and frameworks; an up-to-date knowledge of high-quality, research-based practice in the particular professional discipline, aligned to competent judgement. Commitment to professional codes of conduct and the possession of qualities which foster critical scrutiny of the self in relation to values and attitudes, linked to a capacity for honest reflection, are vital. The development of skill in ethical analysis is a prerequisite for the delivery of high-quality health care.[3]

17.3 MORAL DELIBERATION IN DECISION MAKING

Cognitive processes of deliberation and reflection, which incorporate a number of stages, have been identified as precedents to moral decision making. These include appreciation of the situation and possible outcomes; review of courses of action; selection and application of principles in the final weighing of practical considerations preceding the decision.[5] At consecutive stages, the following points should be borne in mind:

• Each situation should be viewed as unique, pertaining to the individual who is the recipient of care.

- Factual information relevant to the situation should be gathered; disputed facts identified; supporting evidence for the facts critically appraised.
- Courses of action should be formulated and potential outcomes predicted.
- Consideration should be given to resources which could support courses of action; to precedent situations which could illuminate a decision: and to the quantification of risks in relation to harm.
- Moral principles significantly relevant to the particular situation should be identified, that is, rights, duties, benefits, minimising harm and respecting autonomy.
- The interface with the law must be considered and guidance sought from codes of professional conduct.
- Reflection and weighing of principles and consequences which create the most moral outcome should precede the decision to act.

17.4 ETHICAL PRINCIPLES INFORMING DECISION MAKING: A SUMMARY

As discussed in 4.1, autonomy is the capacity to think, decide and act on the basis of such thought and decision, freely and independently.[6] Rational, competent individuals possess the right to choose, accept or reject health care in the exercise of their autonomous will. Respect for the autonomy of an individual in relation to self-determination is justified from the utilitarian perspective, in that the exercise of autonomy, insofar as others are not harmed, will maximise happiness. Mill[7] considered it only justifiable to intervene in the life of another to prevent harm to others. In contrast, Kant's[8] justification for autonomy (see 4.2.2) rests on the maxim to 'act in such a way that you always treat humanity, whether in your own person or in the person of another, never simply as a means, but always at the same time as an end'. As rational agents we should show respect for the autonomy of others in health care decision making, either as recipients of care or as members of the health care team. However, to what extent do individuals wish to exercise their autonomy?

Beneficence and non-maleficence are also key ethical principles (see 5.2) which provide a basis for decision making by the health care professional. Acting for the benefit of individuals to maximise happiness, remove causes of unhappiness and take positive steps to prevent or not to inflict harm can be justified both from consequentialist and deontological perspective (see 4.2.1 and 4.2.2). The Principle of Justice as fairness requires equals to be treated equally (see 6.1) and is another vital consideration in decision making, for example, in facilitating access to health care (see 14.1).

17.5 ETHICAL FRAMEWORKS

A number of ethical frameworks or models which incorporate key principles have been developed to assist moral deliberation. Fry [9] suggests that these are useful, and when utilised with knowledge and appropriate application of ethical theories and principles, can facilitate the development of skills required for decision making. Essentially, their use has been largely confined to teaching health care professionals practical decision-making methods. Relatively few have been described in the nursing literature. Griepp[2] developed a model of decision making based on general systems theory which incorporates concepts and definitions of nurses, clients and the process of nursing. The model is concerned with the potential for psychosociocultural variables on the part of the recipient of care or nurse to inhibit or enhance interactions with others and which may affect the 'rightness' of health care given and received. The ethical framework for this model, which is deontological, is based on the ICN code[10] and ANA professional code[11], which emphasise autonomy, beneficence, non-maleficence, justice and professional accountability. The framework does not incorporate stages in the process of moral deliberation.

In contrast, the ethical grid model developed by Seedhouse and Lovett[3] to teach practical decision-making methods to medical practitioners covers a range of considerations which might affect moral deliberation. The practitioner is required to engage in moral reasoning at four different levels, that is, in relation to the principles behind health work (respect for and creation of autonomy), duties of the health professional (truth telling, non-maleficence), beneficial outcomes for the recipients of care, and external considerations (resources, the law, risks, codes of practice and certainty of evidence available). Its use requires the identification of significant principles relevant to the situation and justification of a course of action. An algorithm subsequently derived from the grid describes five pathways to assist decision making, incorporating external considerations, moral duties, central conditions of health work and consequences, leading into a final common pathway. Necessary decision steps include the assessment of priorities and conflicts. Used in the context of case-study analysis, this is an invaluable approach to the development of decision-making skills.

17.6 FACTORS INFLUENCING DECISION MAKING

A number of social, political and institutional factors may constrain the exercise of respect for autonomy and beneficence by health care professionals (see Chapters 14 and 15). In addition, spiritual beliefs, rights and individual views may influence the extent to which individuals wish to participate in decision making.

17.6.1 Religious influences
Rumbold[12] reviewed the significant influence that cultural and religious factors can have on decisions by health care professionals and patients. For example, in Judaism an imperative obligation exists to preserve and respect life and patients do not have the right to refuse life-saving treatment. Catholicism offers sets of principles derived from theology, from which problem-oriented rules and insights (casuistry) are drawn to help individuals arrive at decisions.[13]

17.6.2 Rights
Historically, individuals have been perceived as passive recipients of care, who were not consulted in the decision-making process. Past views have been encapsulated in the following comments by Gaddow:

'In most professions, those who consult the professional are not capable of making decisions because they are not professionals ... [furthermore] ... persons in need of professional care are incompetent until proved otherwise.'[14]

In recent years, perspectives on the traditional roles of 'patients/client' and, indeed, health care professionals, have changed considerably, with the consumer movement contributing significantly to the active involvement of its proponents in all aspects of health care delivery. This apparent change has been evolved for ethical, social and legal reasons.[15] Predominantly, a shift has occurred from the paternalistic, biomedical model of care to an autonomy model, with its attendant emphasis on the rights of consumers which ensure that individual preferences may not be overridden and are reinforced by legislation. The consumer role has been summarised by Beisecker thus:

> *'... the consumer listens to the thoughts of the provider, but ultimately makes his/her own decision'.[16]*

Effective information giving is crucial to this, so it is not surprising to find that reviews of the research literature also reveal changing patterns in communication related to diagnosis, prognosis and treatment which parallel the rise of consumerism.

For example, Davis and Jameton[17] have shown that the medical literature in the US of 30 years ago demonstrated that most doctors preferred not to tell patients about a diagnosis of cancer, a trend which has now almost completely reversed. Contemporary changes are also reflected in the introduction of the Patient's Charter[18] which requires individuals to be given clear explanations of any proposed treatment, risks and alternatives, before deciding whether or not to agree to treatment. This is only one of ten rights linked to 14 charter standards, which have been developed to improve health service delivery.

Consumers' rights have been equated with active collaboration in care.[19] The WHO[20, 21] has stressed that involvement of recipients in care is not only a right but a duty, and that social and financial considerations reinforce this. For health care professionals, encouraging collaboration in care, professional beneficence can become tainted with cynicism where issues of cost-cutting are strong service motives.

Another important issue in relation to rights is that a right to refuse treatment can generate conflict with the health care professionals' perceived duty to benefit individuals. A controversial question also arises concerning the extent to which individuals may decline to actively participate in health care decisions, or collaborate in care. Is there a moral duty to self, which involves taking responsibility for one's own health? From which decisions, if any, should we be allowed to renounce our rights?

Renunciation of control and lack of involvement in decision making could theoretically diminish some benefits of recovery. For example, in individuals undergoing mastectomy, Morris and Royle[22] have shown that reduced levels of anxiety and depression are experienced in the post-operative period by those who retained control of decision making in considering the treatment options.

17.6.3 Patients' views

Respect for the autonomy of rational agents requires that individuals are informed about their treatment and the possible options for intervention. As Gillon[6] has noted, situations can and do arise where consumers intentionally delegate their autonomy in decision making to doctors.

Provided these individuals are exercising a truly autonomous choice, then respect for autonomy as a moral and professional requirement has been maintained.

However, to what extent do the recipients of care actually wish to be involved in decision making?

Waterworth and Luker[23] investigated this issue in 12 cases using in-depth interviews, based on a grounded theory approach to analysis. Findings from this study suggested that hospitalised individuals were not all keen to participate in decisions concerning their care. Several felt it important to exhibit the 'right' behaviour, to comply with nursing routines, relinquishing freedom and responsibilities in order to toe the line. Waterworth and Luker suggest that some individual's fears of punitive action places enormous responsibility on nurses and midwives not to unwittingly coerce people to comply. A later study by Biley[24], also using open ended interviews, explored the views of individuals following surgery about decision making in nursing aspects of care following discharge. Findings indicated that those who were more severely ill were most willing to relinquish control and delegate decisions about care to nurses. In general, individuals were less concerned with decisions related to medical/surgical procedures or technical aspects of care, but preferred to make decisions in areas where they were confident in knowledge, for example, in activities of daily living. Biley[24] emphasised that individual's views of decision making in nursing, which is principally concerned with 'care' not cure, could differ from their view of medical decisions.

Similar findings have emerged from some medical surveys. For example, Strull[25] found that only 53% of those attending an outpatient medical clinic for hypertension wanted to be involved in the decision making process. A significant number preferred clinicians, whom they perceived as having the appropriate knowledge to make decisions about hypotensive drug therapy. Clearly, it is not possible to generalise such findings from case studies and making comparisons between some investigations is difficult due to differences in the severity of illness and cultural factors inherent in the research design. However, it is evident that health care professionals should not assume that all recipients of care wish to participate in decision making and should be sensitive to the possibility of unwitting, paternalistic coercion, which infringes autonomy. In relation to this Gillon[6] emphasised that a sensitive, skilled practitioner, who respects the individual's autonomy, can elicit information needs and discern the extent to which involvement in decision making is desired. It is important to bear in mind that the extent to which individuals wish or are able to participate in decision making can change during the course of treatment; this should be monitored continuously over time, so that appropriate adjustments to participation can be made.

17.7 CARING – THE CONTEXT OF DECISION MAKING

Ethical decisions are made in the context of 'care' received by individuals, but what is care? Brown et al.[5] define caring as 'to supply concern, protection and preservation', implying the capacity to feel and understand for another person in a situation. Care is explicit in definitions of both medicine and nursing, thus; 'tested knowledge, skills and experience constituting the science and art of care, alleviation and prevention of disease and injury'.[26]

> 'Nursing is.assisting the patient sick or well in the performance of those activities contributing to health or its recovery, that he/she would do unaided, if he/she had the necessary strength, will or knowledge.'[27]

Noddings[28] suggests that 'care involves engrossment and motivational displacement, where the carer sees a situation from the viewpoint of the recipient,' and that a positive mutual regard exists between the carer and recipient. Brown et al.[5] view the ethics of caring as not 'a matter of actions which ought to be done; but to a great extent, an ethics of virtue'. Rhodes[29] suggests that the caring relationship requires specific attributes or virtues to be developed by the carer, including patience, compassion, fortitude, courage, hopefulness, humility, warmth and honesty.

Scrutiny of the contemporary nursing literature on the concept of caring reveals extensive analysis of its attributes, components, professional and lay approaches and relationships to moral reasoning. Olesen[30] suggests that tension exists between the concept of caring and traditional views of justice-based ethics, postulated by Rawls (see 6.3).[31] The notion of justice as fairness incorporates the consideration of parties in a situation as rational and mutually disinterested. Olesen[30] has emphasised that in caring the nurse is not a disinterested party and that the concept of caring can be problematic, because it may include morally irrelevant factors, such as liking and friendship.

Further tensions are apparent in the ethical framework of Kant,[8] based on universal principles (see 2.2.2). Respect for the personhood of others was found by Kant to be a significant limitation to friendship. However, Olesen[30] considers that caring actions are always limited by the universal principle of moral equality of all recipients of care and the concept of duty of care, which take precedence.

17.8 PRACTITIONER–CONSUMER RELATIONSHIPS

In terms of power distribution, the practitioner–consumer relationship is unequal, with the advantage loaded towards the professional carer. Vulnerable recipients of care are disadvantaged by their ill health, the unfamiliar environment and other stressors. Often not at a neutral point in their lives, their capacity for decision-making may be impaired. Advantaged by their scientific knowledge, professional authority and institutional power, the health care practitioner holds the dominant balance in the relationship. However, Kennedy and Grubb[32] emphasised that the ultimate right to know and choose lies with the recipients of care. How can this be facilitated? From a contemporary nursing perspective, Brown et al.[5] view the caring role as one in which recipients of care are assisted to examine their own views and values, and their understanding, informed in an empathetic way. Seedhouse and Lovett[3] have underlined the need for open, liberal, consultative medical practice in which information is shared in the decision-making process. Both professional perspectives agree on the need to avoid strong paternalism, coercion and persuasion.

17.9 NURSE–DOCTOR RELATIONSHIPS

Although nursing and medicine are united in their common purposes of respect for, and service to, humanity, which are enshrined in professional codes of conduct, conflicts can arise. Yarling and McElmurry[33] identified diverse factors, such as paternalism, sexism, a subservient role and position in terms of power, as diminishing nurses' ethical practice, and their capacity to make independent judgements about patient care. Historically, nurses have been viewed as being 'under obligations to carry out the physicians orders'.[34] Brown et al.[5] suggested that professional conflicts can be generated by the espousal of different ethical models of decision making, nurses tending to adhere to an autonomy model and doctors to a beneficence model. Difficulties with the latter can arise where the patient's best interests are interpreted from the medical viewpoint, supporting paternalistic notions that 'doctor knows best' by virtue of their knowledge, expertise and professional authority.[26]

In assuming an advocacy role, nurses may feel that individual's wishes have not been considered, on the basis of incompetence, varying degrees of diminished autonomy or that strong paternalism has been exerted in overriding the views of a person capable of making an autonomous decision. In what situations is conflict likely to arise? Yarling and McElmurry[33] suggested that the most common sources of conflict are generated by decisions regarding pain control, treatment withdrawal, resuscitation and information exchange. However, with the recent unifying movement by all health care professionals towards an autonomy model of decision making in patient care, it is to be hoped that a positive renegotiation and alignment of professional relationships will occur, which will widen involvement in decision making. If health professionals are to function as an efficient team working in collaboration and capable of making effective decisions, then clarification of responsibilities, accountability and clear lines of communication are essential. Effective team operation requires agreement on the moral aims, objectives and policies regarding decisions which will benefit the care of individuals. The promotion of respect for autonomy, a consideration of individuals as ends in themselves and respect for the autonomy of professional colleagues is crucial. Can we achieve this ideal? Time will tell.

LEARNING EXERCISES

1. Define the scope and purpose of moral decision making.
2. With reference to a case study example drawn from your practice, identify the ethical principles which produce a basis for decision making.
3. Describe the attitudes of professional relationships which enhance ethical decision making.
4. How may the autonomy of the patient/client be preserved in treatment decisions?
5. Team ethical decision making: myth or reality? Discuss.

REFERENCES

1. Montaigne, M.E. (1580) *Essays*. Translated by J.M. Cohen (1970). Penguin, Harmondsworth.
2. Griepp, M.E. (1992) 'Griepp's model of ethical decision making'. *Journal of Advanced Nursing*, **17**, 734–8.
3. Seedhouse and Lovett (1992) *Practical Medical Ethics*. John Wiley, Chichester, UK.
4. Levine (1990) 'Nursing Ethics and the Ethical Nurse'. In *Professional Ethics and Nursing*. (Eds. J. Thompson and H. Thompson) Krieger Publishing, Malabar, Florida.
5. Brown, J.M., Kitson, A.L. and McKnight, T. (1992) *Challenges in Caring*. Chapman & Hall, London.
6. Gillon, R. (1986) *Philosophical Medical Ethics*. Churchill Livingstone, Edinburgh.
7. Mill, J.S. *On Liberty*. G. Himmelfarb (ed) (1976). Penguin, London.
8. Kant, I. (1785) *Groundwork of the Metaphysics of Morals*. Translated by M. Gregor (1964). Harper Row, UK.

9. Fry, S. (1989) 'Ethical decision making; Part 1: Selecting a framework'. *Nursing Outlook*, **35**(5), 246.
10. International Council of Nurses (ICN) (1973) *Code for Nurses*. ICN, Geneva.
11. American Nurses Association (1985) *Code for Nursing, Interpretative Statements*. ANA, Missouri.
12. Rumbold (1993) Ethics in Nursing Practice, 2nd Edition. Ballière Tindall.
13. Veatch, R.M. (1981) *A Theory of Medical Ethics*. Basic Books, New York.
14. Gaddow, S. (1989) 'An ethical case for patient self-determination'. *Seminars in Oncology Nursing*, **5**(2), 99–101.
15. Sutherland, H.J., Llewellyn-Thomas, H.A., Lockwood, G.A., *et al.* (1989) 'Cancer patients: their desire for information and participation in treatment decisions?' *Journal of the Royal Society of Medicine*, **82**, 260–3.
16. Beisecker, A.E. (1988) 'Ageing and the desire for information and input in medical decisions; patient consumerism in medical encounters'. *The Gerontologist*, **28**(3), 330–5.
17. Davis, A.J. and Jameton, A. (1987) 'Nursing and medical students' attitudes towards nursing, disclosure of information to patients; a pilot study'. *Journal of Advanced Nursing*, **12**, 691–8.
18. Department of Health (1992) *The Patient's Charter: A Summary*. HMSO, London.
19. Teasdale, K. (1987) 'Partnership with Patients?' *Professional Nurse* **2**(12):397–399.
20. World Health Organisation (WHO) (1979) *Formulating Strategies for Health by the Year 2000*. WHO, Geneva.
21. WHO (1984) 'Health Education in Self Care: Possibilities and Limitations'. *WHO Newsletter* 1(2):5–7.
22. Morris, J. and Royle, G.T. (1988) 'Offering Patients a Choice of Surgery for Early Breast Cancer'. *Social Science Medicine*. **26**(6):583–585.
23. Waterworth, S. and Luker, H.A. (1990) 'Reluctant collaborators; do patients want to be involved in decisions concerning care?' *Journal of Advanced Nursing*, **15**, 971–6.
24. Biley, F.C. (1992) 'Some determinants that effect patient participation in decision making about nursing care'. *Journal of Advanced Nursing*, **17**, 414–21.
25. Strull, W.M., Lo, B. and Charles, G. (1984) 'Do patients want to participate in medical decision making?' *Journal of the American Medical Association*, **252**(21), 2990–4.
26. Beauchamp, T. and McCullough, L. (1984) *Medical Ethics: The Moral Responsibility of Physicians*. Prentice Hall, New Jersey, USA.
27. Henderson, V. (1966) *The Nature of Nursing; A Definition and its Implications, Practice, Research and Education*. Macmillan Press, New York.
28. Noddings, N. (1984) *Caring*. University of California Press, California.
29. Rhodes, M.L. (1986) *Ethical Dilemma in Social work Practice*. Routledge & Keegan Paul, London.
30 Olesen, D.P. (1992) 'Controversies in nursing ethics: a historical review'. *Journal of Advanced Nursing*, **12**, 1020–7.
31. Rawls, J (1971) *A Theory of Justice*. Harvard University Press, USA.
32. Kennedy, I. and Grubb, A. (1989) *Medical law, Texts and Materials*. Butterworth, London.
33. Yarling, R.R. and McElmurry, B.J. (1986) 'The moral foundations of nursing'. *Advances in Nursing Science*, **8**(2), 63–73.
34. ICN (1965) *Code for Nurses*. ICN, Geneva.

Key points

- The Principle of Autonomy. In certain areas an individual has a right to be self-governing.
- The Principle of Beneficence. The well-being or benefit of the individual ought to be promoted.
- The Principle of Non-maleficence. One ought to do no harm.
- Consequentialism. There is one ultimate moral aim, that outcomes be as good as possible.
- Deontology. Certain prima facie duties such as truth-telling, non-maleficence, justice, and beneficence are morally obligatory.
- The Principle of Justice. Equals ought to be considered equally.
- Strong paternalism; limiting or denying freedom of choice to a competent person capable of making an autonomous decision.

APPENDIX A

Glossary of Philosophical and Health Care Terms

Abortion Termination of pregnancy.

Accountability The extent to which health care professionals can be held in law to account for their actions; making judgements in relation to actions which have measurable outcomes.

Advocacy Defending the cause of an individual or group; informing patients of their rights in health care decisions.

AIDS Acquired immune deficiency syndrome caused by infection with the HIV virus.

Amniocentesis A diagnostic procedure in which amniotic fluid is withdrawn from the sac surrounding a fetus. Down's syndrome and other genetic disorders can be identified by examination of the fluid.

Anencephalic Absence of the brain and part of the skull at birth.

Autonomy The capacity to think, to decide and then to act on the basis of such thought and decision freely and independently.

Autonomy, Principle of In certain areas, an individual has a right to be self-governing.

Beneficence, Principle of The well-being or benefit of the individual ought to be promoted.

Caesarean section Delivery of a baby through a surgical incision in the abdominal and uterine walls.

Categorical imperative (Kant) Act only on the maxim through which you can at the same time will that it should become a universal law.

Chemotherapy Treatment of different types of cancer or infections using specific drugs, that is, anti-cancer drugs and antibiotics, respectively.

Cognitivism Moral judgements are statements that are capable of being true or false.

Confidentiality Non-disclosure of information given in confidence.

Consequentialism Outcomes be as good as possible.
- **Act consequentialism** An action is right if it produces the best outcome possible.
- **Hedonistic consequentialism (utilitarianism)** Actions are right in proportion as they promote happiness.
- **Interest or Preference Consequentialism** Actions are right in proportion as they promote interest or preference satisfaction.
- **Rule Consequentialism** A rule is right if it produces the best outcome possible.

Coronary artery bypass grafting Surgical insertion of a vein graft to bypass the narrowed, diseased area of a coronary artery.

Craniotomy Removal of part of the skull (cranium).

Declining Marginal Utility, Principle of For a given individual, a set amount of something is more useful when that individual has little of it than when he or she has a lot.

Diabetes mellitus A disorder characterised by an absolute or relative lack of the hormone insulin, resulting in abnormalities of glucose, fat and protein metabolism.

Doctrine of the Double Effect There is a difference between what one aims at (one's direct intention) and what is foreseen but is not intended (one's oblique intention).

Down's syndrome A genetic disorder characterised by the possession of 47 instead of 46 (the norm) chromosomes resulting in mental handicap and distinctive physical features.

Embryo The developing baby during the first eight weeks following conception.

Epilepsy A condition resulting in abnormal electrical activity in the brain, characterised by fits.

Euthanasia A deliberate death brought about by one person for the benefit of another person, the person whose life is taken.
- **Involuntary euthanasia** Euthanasia where the individual has not requested it but it is thought to be in that individual's best interests.
- **Non-voluntary euthanasia** Euthanasia where the individual has no views about the continuation of their life because they are not capable of understanding the choice between life and death.
- **Voluntary euthanasia** Euthanasia in response to an individual's request.

Fetus A developing child from the end of the eighth week following conception until birth at 40 weeks.

Hypoglycaemia A low concentration of blood glucose: <2.5 mmol per litre (abnormal)

Hypothermia A decline in body temperature below 35°C which may lead to impaired consciousness or death.

Hypovolaemic shock Shock caused by a low circulating blood volume, typically caused by haemorrhage.

Informed consent A voluntary agreement to undergo treatment made by a competent person on the basis of adequate information and without coercion.

Justice, Principle of Equals ought to be considered equally.

Laparoscopy Examination of the interior of the abdomen using a fibre-optic endoscope to view the gut or reproductive tract.

Metastasis A secondary malignant tumour generated from a primary cancer.

Multiple sclerosis Disease of the central nervous system associated with demyelination of nerve fibres and characterised by variable disabilities affecting neurological function.

Non-maleficence, Principle of One ought to do no harm.

Paternalism Refusing to accede in another person's autonomous choices for that person's benefit.

Persistent vegetative state (PVS) A state resulting from acute brain damage in which function of the cerebral cortex is permanently lost.

'Persons' Rational beings aware of their existence over time (self-conscious).

Quality adjusted life year (QALY) A measure of life enhancing and extending aspects of treatment. For a given medical condition the QALY value is the number of QALYs experienced with treatment minus the number if left untreated.

Senile dementia A condition in which mental ability declines in an individual over 65 years of age. In most cases, the cause is cerebrovascular disease.

Sentient Possession of sensation.

Ultrasound scan A non-invasive diagnostic technique using high-frequency sound waves to visualise internal body structures.

Ventilator Mechanical device to provide artificial ventilation of an individual who lacks the ability to breathe normally.

Zygote A fertilised egg consisting of a single cell.

APPENDIX B

The Hippocratic Oath

I swear by Apollo the physician, and Aesculapius and Health, and All-hel, and all the gods and goddesses, that, according to my ability and judgement, I will keep this Oath and this stipulation - to reckon him who taught me this Art equally dear to me as my parents, to share my substance with him, and relieve his necessities if required; to look upon his offspring in the same footing as my own brothers, and to teach them this Art, if they shall wish to learn it, without fee or stipulation; and that by percept, lecture and every other mode of instruction, I will impart a knowledge of the Art to my own sons, and those of my teachers, and to disciples bound by a stipulation and oath according to the law of medicine, but to none other. I will follow that system of regimen which, according to my ability and judgement, I consider for the benefit of my patients, and abstain from whatever is deleterious and mischievous. I will give no deadly medicine to anyone if asked, nor suggest any such counsel; and in like manner I will not give to a woman a pessary to produce abortion. With purity and with holiness I will pass my life and practise my Art. I will not cut persons labouring under the stone, but will leave this to be done by men who are practitioners of this work. Into whatever houses I enter, I will go into them for the benefit of the sick, and will abstain from every voluntary act of mischief and corruption; and, further, from the seduction of females, or males, of freemen or slaves. Whatever, in connection with my professional practice, not in connection with it, I see or hear, in the life of men, which ought not to be spoken of abroad, I will not divulge, as reckoning that all such should be kept secret. While I continue to keep this Oath unviolated, may it be granted to me to enjoy life and the practice of the Art, respected by all men, in all times. But should I trespass and violate this Oath, may the reverse be my lot.

APPENDIX C

International Code of Medical Ethics

AT THE TIME OF BEING ADMITTED AS A MEMBER OF THE MEDICAL PROFESSION:

I solemnly pledge myself to consecrate my life to the service of humanity;

I will give to my teachers the respect and gratitude which is their due;

I will practise my profession with conscience and dignity;

The health of my patient will be my first consideration;

I will respect the secrets which are confided in me, even after the patient has died;
I will maintain by all the means in my power, the honour and the noble traditions
of the medical profession;

My colleagues will be my brothers;

I will not permit considerations of religion, nationality, race, party politics or social
standing to intervene between my duty and my patients;

I will maintain the utmost respect for human life from its beginning even under threat
and I will not use my medical knowledge contrary to the laws of humanity;

I make these promises solemnly, freely and upon my honour.

The English text of the International Code of Medical Ethics is as follows:

Duties of physicians in general

A PHYSICIAN SHALL always maintain the highest standards of professional conduct.

A PHYSICIAN SHALL not permit motives of profit to influence the free and
independent exercise of professional judgement on behalf of patients.

A PHYSICIAN SHALL, in all types of medical practice, be dedicated to providing
competent medical service in full technical and moral independence, with
compassion and respect for human dignity.

A PHYSICIAN SHALL deal honestly with patients and colleagues, and strive to expose
those physicians deficient in character or competence, or who engage in fraud or
deception.

THE FOLLOWING PRACTICES ARE DEEMED TO BE UNETHICAL CONDUCT:

a) Self advertising by physicians, unless permitted by the laws of the country and the Code of Ethics of the national medical association.

b) Paying or receiving any fee or any other consideration solely to procure the referral of a patient or for prescribing or referring a patient to any source.

A PHYSICIAN SHALL respect the rights of patients, of colleagues and of any other health professionals, and shall safeguard patient confidences.

A PHYSICIAN SHALL act only in the patient's interest when providing medical care which might have the effect of weakening the physical and mental condition of the patient.

A PHYSICIAN SHALL use great caution in divulging discoveries or new techniques or treatment through non-professional channels.

A PHYSICIAN SHALL certify only that which he has personally verified.

Duties of physicians to the sick

A PHYSICIAN SHALL always bear in mind the obligation of preserving human life.

A PHYSICIAN SHALL owe his patients complete loyalty and all the resources of his science. Whenever an examination or treatment is beyond the physician's capacity he should summon another physician who has the necessary ability.

A PHYSICIAN SHALL preserve absolute confidentiality on all he knows about his patient even after the patient has died.

A PHYSICIAN SHALL give emergency care as a humanitarian duty unless he is assured that others are willing and able to give such care.

Duties of physicians to each other

A PHYSICIAN SHALL behave towards his colleagues as he would have them behave towards him.

A PHYSICIAN SHALL NOT entice patients from his colleagues.

A PHYSICIAN SHALL observe the principles of "The Declaration of Geneva" approved by the World Medical Association.

APPENDIX D

Declaration of Helsinki

HUMAN EXPERIMENTATION

It is the mission of the medical doctor to safeguard the health of the people. His or her knowledge and conscience are dedicated to the fulfilment of this mission.

The Declaration of Geneva of the World Medical Association binds the physician with the words, "The health of my patient will be my first consideration", and the International Code of Medical Ethics declares that "A physician shall act only in the patient's interest when providing medical care which might have the effect of weakening the physical and mental condition of the patient".

The purpose of biomedical research involving human subjects must be to improve diagnostic, therapeutic and prophylactic procedures and the understanding of the aetiology and pathogenesis of disease.

In current medical practice most diagnostic, therapeutic or prophylactic procedures involve hazards. This applies especially to biomedical research.

Medical progress is based on research which ultimately must rest in part on experimentation involving human subjects.

In the field of biomedical research a fundamental distinction must be recognised between medical research in which the aim is essentially diagnostic or therapeutic for a patient, and medical research, the essential object of which is purely scientific and without implying direct diagnostic or therapeutic value to the person subjected to the research.

Special caution must be exercised in the conduct of research which may affect the environment, and the welfare of animals used for research must be respected.

I Basic principles

1 Biomedical research involving human subjects must conform to generally accepted scientific principles and should be based on adequately performed laboratory and animal experimentation and a thorough knowledge of the scientific literature.

2. The design and performance of each experimental procedure involving human subjects should be clearly formulated in an experimental protocol which should be transmitted to a specially appointed independent committee for consideration, comment and guidance.

3. Biomedical research involving human subjects should be conducted only by scientifically qualified persons and under the supervision of a clinically competent medical person. The responsibility for the human subject must always rest with the medically qualified person and never rest on the subject of the research, even though the subject has given his or her consent.

4. Biomedical research involving human subjects cannot legitimately be carried out unless the importance of the objective is in proportion to the inherent risk to the subject.

5. Every biochemical research project involving human subjects should be preceded by careful assessment of predictable risks in comparison with foreseeable benefits to

the subject or to others. Concern for the interests of the subject must always prevail over the interest of science and society.

6. The right of the research subject to safeguard his or her integrity must always be respected. Every precaution should be taken to respect the privacy of the subject and to minimize the impact of the study on the subject's physical and mental integrity and on the personality of the subject.

7. Physicians should abstain from engaging in research projects involving human subjects unless they are satisfied that the hazards involved are believed to be predictable. Physicians should cease any investigation if the hazards are found to outweigh the potential benefits.

8. In publication of the results of his or her research, the physician is obliged to preserve the accuracy of the results. Reports of experimentation not in accordance with the principles laid down in this Declaration should not be accepted for publication.

9. In any research on human beings, each potential subject must be adequately informed of the aims, methods, anticipated benefits and potential hazards of the study and the discomfort it may entail. He or she should be informed that he or she is at liberty to abstain from participation in the study and that he or she is free to withdraw his or her consent to participation at any time. The physician should then obtain the subject's freely-given informed consent, preferably in writing.

10. When obtaining informed consent for the research project the physician should be particularly cautious if the subject is in a dependent relationship to him or her or may consent under duress. In that case the informed consent should be obtained by a physician who is not engaged in the investigation and who is completely independent of this official relationship.

11. In case of legal incompetence, informed consent should be obtained from the legal guardian in accordance with national legislation. Where physical or mental incapacity makes it impossible to obtain informed consent, or when the subject is a minor, permission from the responsible relative replaces that of the subject in accordance with national legislation. Whenever the minor child is in fact able to give a consent, the minor's consent must be obtained in addition to the consent of the minor's legal guardian.

12. The research protocol should always contain a statement of the ethical considerations involved and should indicate that the principles enunciated in the present Declaration are complied with.

II Medical research combined with professional care
(Clinical research)

1. In the treatment of the sick person, the physician must be free to use a new diagnostic and therapeutic measure, if in his or her judgement it offers hope of saving life, re-establishing health or alleviating suffering.

2. The potential benefits, hazards and discomfort of a new method should be weighed against the advantages of the best current diagnostic and therapeutic methods.

3. In any medical study, every patient - including those of a control group, if any - should be assured of the best proven diagnostic and therapeutic method.

4. The refusal of the patient to participate in a study must never interfere with the physician-patient relationship.

5. If the physician considers it essential not to obtain informed consent, the specific reasons for this proposal should be stated in the experimental protocol for transmission to the independent committee (I.2).

6. The physician can combine medical research with professional care, the objective being the acquisition of new medical knowledge, only to the extent that medical research is justified by its potential diagnostic or therapeutic value for the patient.

III Non-therapeutic biomedical research involving human subjects

(Non-clinical biomedical research)

1. In the purely scientific application of medical research carried out on a human being, it is the duty of the physician to remain the protector of the life and health of that person on whom biomedical research is being carried out.

2. The subjects should be volunteers - either healthy persons or patients for whom the experimental design is not related to the patient's illness.

3. The investigator or the investigating team should discontinue the research if in his/her or their judgement it may, if continued, be harmful to the individual.

4. In research on man, the interest of science and society should never take precedence over considerations related to the wellbeing of the subject.

APPENDIX E

Code of Professional Conduct for the Nurse, Midwife and Health Visitor (June 1992)

EACH REGISTERED NURSE, MIDWIFE AND HEALTH VISITOR SHALL ACT, AT ALL TIMES, IN SUCH A MANNER AS TO:

- safeguard and promote the interests of individual patients and clients;

- serve the interests of society;

- justify public trust and confidence and

- uphold and enhance the good standing and reputation of the professions.

As a registered nurse, midwife or health visitor, you are personally accountable for your practice and, in the exercise of your professional accountability, must:

1. Act always in such a manner as to promote and safeguard the interests and well-being of patients and clients.

2. Ensure that no action or omission on your part, or within your sphere of responsibility, is detrimental to the interests, condition or safety of patients and clients.

3. Maintain and improve your professional knowledge and competence.

4. Acknowledge any limitations in your knowledge and competence and decline any duties or responsibilities unless able to perform them in a safe and skilled manner.

5. Work in an open and co-operative manner with patients, clients and their families, foster their independence and recognise and respect their involvement in the planning and delivery of care.

6. Work in a collaborative and co-operative manner with health care professionals and others involved in providing care, and recognise and respect their particular contributions within the care team.

7. Recognise and respect the uniqueness and dignity of each patient and client, and respond to their need for care, irrespective of their ethnic origin, religious beliefs, personal attributes, the nature of their health problems or any other factor.

8. Report to an appropriate person or authority, at the earliest possible time, any conscientious objection which may be relevant to your professional practice.

9. Avoid any abuse of your privileged relationship with patients and clients and of the privileged access allowed to their person, property, residence or workplace.

10. Protect all confidential information concerning patients and clients obtained in the course of professional practice and make disclosures only with consent, where required by the order of a court or where you can justify disclosure in the wider public interest.

11. Report to an appropriate person or authority, having regard to the physical, psychological and social effects on patients and clients, any circumstances in the environment of care which could jeopardise standards of practice.

12. Report to an appropriate person or authority any circumstances in which safe and appropriate care for patients and clients cannot be provided.

13. Report to an appropriate person or authority where it appears that the health or safety of colleagues is at risk, as such circumstances my compromise standards of practice and care.

14. Assist professional colleagues, in the context of your own knowledge, experience and sphere of responsibility, to develop their professional competence, and assist others in the care team, including informal carers, to contribute safely and to a degree appropriate to their roles.

15. Refuse any gift, favour or hospitality from patients or clients currently in your care which might be interpreted as seeking to exert influence to obtain preferential consideration.

16. Ensure that your registration status is not used in the promotion of commercial products or services, declare any financial or other interests in relevant organisations providing such goods or services and ensure that your professional judgement is not influenced by any commercial considerations.

Reproduced by kind permission of the UKCC.

APPENDIX F

Rules of Professional Conduct for Physiotherapists

1. SCOPE OF PRACTICE
Chartered physiotherapists shall confine themselves to clinical diagnosis and practice in those fields of physiotherapy in which they have been trained and which are recognised by the profession to be beneficial.

The term 'clinical diagnosis' in this rule is intended to establish that a Chartered physiotherapist may, by taking a history and conducting a clinical examination and a functional assessment, come to a conclusion as to the cause of a patient's symptoms and thus justify institution of appropriate physiotherapy.

It does not restrict the extension of appropriate professional skills and practice.

Chartered physiotherapists shall recognise not only the responsibilities but also the limitations of their professional practice. When the recognition of practice is in question, it will be referred to The Chartered Society of Physiotherapy.

Training is defined as the accumulation of knowledge and skills gained by formal education and by experience evaluated at a level of competence acceptable for independent clinical practice.

This rule incorporates the ethical principle defining the relationship between Chartered physiotherapists and patients; i.e. Chartered physiotherapists should always aim to benefit patients through the exercise of their professional knowledge and skills acquired through training and experience. The term 'patient' is used throughout these rules to describe a person receiving the services of a Chartered physiotherapist in the context of preventive, primary or secondary health care provision.

2. RELATIONSHIPS WITH PATIENTS
Chartered physiotherapists shall respect the rights, dignity and individual sensibilities of all their patients.

This rule is intended to define the relationship between Chartered physiotherapists and patients on a basis of mutual trust and respect.

In detail this means that all patients will be treated with courtesy and consideration; they will be informed about and must be given the opportunity to consent to or to decline treatment proposals. This requirement for informed consent also extends to the inclusion of patients in any research activities, which also requires the approval of an ethical committee.

Information as to risk and the options of alternative treatment including any warnings of inherent risks in a procedure must take account of the mental, emotional and physical state of the patient.

Failure to warn a patient of the risks inherent in a procedure which is recommended may constitute a failure to respect the patient's right to make his own decision.

The dignity and feelings of the individual patient shall be uppermost in the mind of the Chartered physiotherapist at all times.

3. RELATIONSHIPS WITH MEDICAL COLLEAGUES

Chartered physiotherapists shall communicate and co-operate with registered medical practitioners in the diagnosis, treatment and management of patients.

This rule does not restrict those Chartered physiotherapists who so wish from accepting the responsibility of independent professional practice. It emphasises that full professional responsibility necessitates keeping patients' doctors appropriately informed and requires effective inter-professional communication to be established in the best interests of patients.

4. RELATIONSHIPS BETWEEN PROFESSIONALS AND WITH CARERS

Chartered physiotherapists shall communicate and co-operate with other health and allied professionals and all others caring for the patient, in the interests of the patient.

It is important that Chartered physiotherapists co-operate appropriately with all those working for the good of the patient. Such co-operation should be an active process, and includes making inter-professional referrals where these are appropriate.

Where any doubt exists as to the credentials of other practitioners involved in the care of patients, verification of their professional status must be obtained.

5. RELATIONSHIPS WITHIN THE PROFESSION

Chartered physiotherapists shall communicate and co-operate with each other and avoid public criticism of colleagues.

This rule is intended to protect patients from becoming the victims of disagreements within the profession which may bring the good name of the profession into disrepute.

6. CONFIDENTIALITY

Chartered physiotherapists shall treat as confidential information obtained by them during the course of the practice of their profession.

This rule is intended to guide members on their responsibilities in relation to the confidentiality of information gained by them in the course of their practice.

This information is not to be divulged to a third party without the written consent of the patient unless the Chartered physiotherapist is directed to do so by a competent legal authority, such as a judge, and unless it is necessary to protect the welfare of the patient and the community.

However, in the context of the medical management of patients, there are occasions when information may be given to the Chartered physiotherapist by patients because of the relationship which exists between them. In such cases, the position must be explained to the patients and their permission requested to pass on what is relevant or vital.

This rule also applies to any information that is obtained during a research project, or clinical examination or peer review procedure, which identifies individual patients, unless written consent is obtained.

Should at any time Chartered physiotherapists breach confidentiality for whatever reason, they must be prepared to justify their actions under this rule.

7. ADVERTISING

Advertising by Chartered physiotherapists in respect of professional activities shall be accurate and professionally restrained.

Because of the importance of the maintenance of the patient/therapist relationship, it is unethical to appeal in person to potential patients, whether such appeals are made face-to-face or by telephone.

Advertisements, whether written or audio-visual, should not be false, fraudulent, misleading, deceptive, self-laudatory, unfair or sensational. This also applies to the use of qualifications and titles. Specific claims should not be made in respect of superiority of personal professional practice, nor of specialist status as a physiotherapist. It is undesirable (but not unethical) to use too many qualifications. Three are usually enough.

While it is right for Chartered physiotherapists to publicise the profession and the practice of physiotherapy, they should act in a restrained manner in respect of their personal practice.

8. SALE OF GOODS

Chartered physiotherapists shall not sell, supply, endorse or promote the sale of goods in ways which exploit their professional relationship with individual patients.

Chartered physiotherapists shouls only sell or supply goods in clinical practice after they have satisfied themselves that the item in question is appropriate to the individual patient's condition. Any handling charge on the sale of goods should be reasonable. Chartered physiotherapists should not accept commission from a third party for recommending, in clinical practice, the purchase of goods.

9. PERSONAL AND PROFESSIONAL STANDARDS

Chartered physiotherapists shall adhere at all times to personal and professional standards which reflect credit on the profession.

This rule has been deliberately framed as a general statement, recognising that it is impossible to specify in precise terms all those actions which could be deemed to amount to professional misconduct now and in the future. It is for the profession itself to determine what, at any particular time, constitutes conduct requiring disciplinary action by the Chartered Society.

The following provides an indication of the types of incidents which would be likely to be brought to the attention of the Chartered Society.

9. (1) Conviction by a Court

Any conviction of a member by a court of law is capable of reflecting adversely on the profession. It is therefore appropriate that the Society should have authority to consider all the circumstances leading to such a conviction and to determine whether disciplinary action by the Society is appropriate.

There will obviously be cases of a minor and/or personal nature where no action by the Chartered Society is required. When such cases are drawn to the Chartered Society's attention, they will normally be dealt with informally.

It is important that a member who is charged with a criminal offence should not plead guilty if he believes he has a defence, since the acceptance of such a guilty plea would be likely to lead to a conviction, and thus bring the member within the jurisdiction of the Chartered Society.

9. (2) Disciplinary Procedure by the State Registration Board

Disciplinary procedures by the State Registration Board resulting in a finding of infamous conduct may be reported to the Chartered Society and may render a member liable to disciplinary proceedings in line with the Society's own regulations.

9. (3) Disciplinary Proceedings by an Employer

Disciplinary proceedings by an employer leading to dismissal from employment will bring a member within the jurisdiction of the Chartered Society. This applies even if the member has been involved in related court proceedings which have not resulted in conviction.

Disciplinary proceedings by an employer leading to punishment short of dismissal (e.g. reprimand) will not normally give rise to disciplinary action by the Chartered Society unless the circumstances are sufficient to found a complaint under another section of the Rules of Professional Conduct.

9. (4) Neglect of Professional Responsibility to a Patient

Examples of neglect of professional responsibility which would be likely to lead to disciplinary action by the Chartered Society are: failure to provide or arrange appropriate treatment; improper delegation of treatment to unqualified helpers; and attempting to carry out procedures or administer drugs in respect of which the member does not have the necessary authority, training or skill.

9. (5) Abuse of Professional Privilege or Skills

The Chartered physiotherapist is privileged to have physical contact with the patient, and to enter the patient's home to administer any advice or course of treatment. Abuse of these privileges for personal reward or satisfaction amounts to a serious breach of the Rules of Professional Conduct. Any attempt to exercise undue influence over the patient in order to obtain personal benefit would be liable to give ground for a complaint to the Chartered Society.

9. (6) Personal Conduct Derogatory to the Reputation of the Profession

Personal conduct which does not lead to conviction by a court of law or disciplinary action by an employer may give rise to disciplinary action by the Chartered Society if such conduct is judged to be derogatory to the reputation of the profession.

Examples are personal misuse or abuse of alcohol or drugs, dishonesty, and indecent or violent behaviour.

Reproduced by the kind permission of the Chartered Society of Physiotherapists, Autumn 1992.

APPENDIX G

Rules of Professional Conduct for Occupational Therapists

A. RELATIONSHIPS WITH, AND RESPONSIBILITIES TO, CONSUMERS

Principle
1. Confidentiality
Beyond any essential sharing of information with professional colleagues, occupational therapists must safeguard confidential information relating to consumers.

Notes
a) The disclosure of confidential information is permissible when :
(i) there is legal compulsion;
(ii) a consumer gives consent;
(iii) as a citizen it is one's duty to act in the public interest.
b) Refer to current NHS Code of Practice on access to personal health information particularly related to Data Protection Act 1984.
c) Refer to Director of Social Services/Social Work for current procedures

i) Contacts made for or on behalf of consumers during the course of treatment will only be made with the consumer's knowledge. Every effort must be made to ensure the consumer is aware of the course of treatment and has given consent to contact being made, particularly with outside agencies.

ii) No information will be given to a consumer (or that person's relatives) about another consumer without the consumer's consent. This principle should also apply to confidences given between colleagues.

iii) Requests from third parties (e.g. solicitors) for information regarding a consumer's diagnosis, treatment, prognosis or future requirements will only be given with (a) the consumer's consent, (b) the consent of the consultant in charge and (c) after clearance from the employing authority's legal advisor. Notes should not be surrendered but an appropriate precis made of the relevant facts. Requests/demands for the notes on a consumer should be directed via the unit general manager or director of Social Services/ Social Work.
iv) All notes shall be kept in a secure place and made available only to those who have a legitimate need to see them. Consumers' requests to see their notes should only be granted when confirmation has been received from all those who have contributed to them that they are happy for this to occur. Access to notes by consumers must conform to the employing authority's procedure.

Principle
2. Cruelty
Occupational therapists must not engage in, or condone, behaviour that causes unnecessary mental or physical distress.

Notes
a) Such behaviour would include an indifference to the pain and misery of others, excessive strictness and instances of inattention or carelessness.
b) Occupational therapists have a duty to use the appropriate means and recognised channels to report, to the appropriate authority, behaviour or action that is indefensible for the unnecessary offence it inflicts upon a consumer.

i) Any treatment that is likely to cause pain or distress should be explained to the consumer before being undertaken and the consumer given the opportunity to refuse it, within his her ability to comprehend.

ii) No occupational therapist shall leave a consumer in pain or distress after treatment, until every effort has been made to alleviate it, or the consumer has been given the opportunity to deal with it. If distress continues, this should be communicated appropriately to relevant other parties.

iii) Any occupational therapist who witnesses or has evidence of treatment, which appears to inflict unnecessary or avoidable pain or distress e.g. bruising, should make this known to his/her head occupational therapist immediately. Where it is appropriate the occupational therapist should intervene within the limits of his her professional competence in an effort to prevent the action continuing.

iv) The head occupational therapist should investigate the situation and seek urgent discussion with the appropriate head of department.

Principle
3. Personal relationships
Occupational therapists must refrain in the course of their professional work, from entering into personal relationships which disrupt treatment and/or family life, or otherwise damage professional trust.

Notes
a) It is inevitable that occupational therapists might experience strong positive or negative feelings towards consumers. These should never be allowed to affect treatment. When necessary, consideration should be given to a change of therapist.
b) Occasions will arise when occupational therapists will already know or will want to enter into a friendship with a consumer. The professional relationship need not be damaged if therapists define the boundaries between personal and working environments and always respect these.

i) If a therapist has or develops a personal friendship with a consumer during his/her treatment, this should be made known to the supervising occupational therapist who should then ensure that the treatment of the consumer by the occupational therapist is not in any way affected.

ii) If an occupational therapist experiences excessively negative feelings towards a consumer or feels that the clash of personalities in some way impedes treatment, this should be made known to the supervising occupational therapist. The supervisor should then work with the occupational therapist to see if it is possible for the relationship to be improved. If it is not possible then another therapist should be assigned to that consumer.

Principle
4 Respecting consumers' rights
Occupational therapists have a responsibility to promote and protect the dignity, privacy, autonomy and safety of all consumers with whom they come into contact.

Notes
a) Occupational therapists must be aware of local procedures and use these in a manner which promotes privacy, dignity, autonomy and safety.
b) Protecting privacy might extend to safeguards when publishing visual or written material. Refer to local procedure.
c) Occupational therapists must observe the provisions of the Mental Health Acts and the Health and Safety at Work Acts as they apply to the United Kingdom.

i) All consumers will be treated with respect and in a manner which retains their own personal dignity.

ii) Consumers should always be encouraged to participate in the decision about their treatment and further management.

iii) Consumers should always have the treatment offered by occupational therapists explained to them and the therapist should ensure that this is understood in so far as the consumer is able. Consumers have a right to refuse treatment and it should be respected. This should be reported to the doctor concerned.

iv) All adult consumers will be addressed formally as Mr/Mrs/Miss etc. unless they indicate a wish or agree to be called by their forenames. In the case of children, forenames can be used or a name by which they have chosen to be called. If the convention of the ward/unit is to use forenames, this should be followed if it is seen as appropriate in the circumstances and retains the consumer's dignity.

v) No conversation about a consumer shall be held in a location or manner where these can be overheard. Discussions about a consumer held within his/her hearing should include him/her.
vi) Wherever possible, discussions/conversations with consumers about private or personal issues should be held in a location which cannot be overheard by other consumers.

Principle
5. Maintenance of service to consumers
The occupational therapist must identify and strive to maintain priority areas of service during manpower shortage, financial restriction, and industrial disputes. Liaison with other professionals is essential to ensure consumers' needs are met as far as possible. Occupational therapists have a right to state and support their views

about the service for which they work, but should avoid any action which places the consumer at risk.

Notes
a) When establishing priorities, a balance must be struck between the needs of the consumers and the competence, knowledge, training and experience of the available staff.
b) No action should be taken which affects consumers whose ultimate safety might be at risk. This would include services to high dependency consumers which, if withdrawn, would cause severe hardship.
c) Further guidance should be sought in the following sequence
i) local manager
ii) local steward
iii) British Association of Occupational Therapists' Council representative
iv) British Association of Occupational Therapists' headquarters.

i) An action which will affect the service to consumers must be discussed with the head occupational therapist who will in turn discuss with the district/area occupational therapist, or local authority equivalents.

ii) Occupational therapists have a duty of care to consumers whom they accept for treatment. Every consumer should have a clearly recorded assessment of need and objectives of treatment. At times of staff shortage, financial restriction, or industrial action, this recorded assessment of need should also clearly state those objectives that have to be achieved in order to maintain a minimum level of satisfactory occupational therapy service. If the therapist feels unable to reach these minimum standards, then this should be notified immediately to the head occupational therapist who will, after discussion with the relevant people, determine what action is to be taken.

iii) Head occupational therapists and supervising occupational therapists who are operating a minimally acceptable level of service should notify this, in writing, on a regular basis to their unit general manager and the district/area occupational therapist or local authority equivalents. This notification should include statistics of waiting lists and unallocated or incompleted work.

iv) Where problems persist, the head occupational therapist must assess the priorities of service delivery and discuss with the district/area occupational therapist areas for withdrawal of occupational therapy services. The head occupational therapist and/or the district/area occupational therapist will discuss the agreed areas with his/her designated manager or director of Social Services.

B. PROFESSIONAL INTEGRITY

Principle
6. Personal integrity
The highest standards of personal integrity are expected of occupational therapists. They must not engage in any criminal activity in the practice of their profession.

Notes

The establishment and maintenance of professional integrity will be dependent on the interpersonal trust created by occupational therapists with colleagues and consumers. The qualities of fairness, honesty, consistency and truthfulness, combined with the use of discretion will enable such trust to develop.

i) Occupational therapists must not only act in accordance with the highest level of personal integrity but be seen to do so.
Local arrangements for the handling of money, dealing with consumer's effects etc. are available in occupational therapy departments and must be followed.

ii) Arrangements made with consumers or their relatives or with other personnel must always be kept, or if this proves impossible, a satisfactory and honest reason given.

iii) Errors made or arrangements not kept, where no damage occurs to the customer, should be rectified as soon as possible and an apology made. Where an error could be construed as negligence, the wording of any communication should be discussed with the head occupational therapist and/or district area occupational therapist before any response is made.

Principle
7. Discrimination
Occupational therapists must not discriminate against consumers on the basis of race, colour, handicap, national origin, age, gender, sexual preference, religion, political beliefs or status in society.

Principle
8. Toxic substances
Occupational therapists must not be under the influence of any toxic substance which impairs the performance of their duties.
   Occupational therapists must not encourage others in the misuse of toxic substances.

Notes

Misuse of alcohol, drugs or solvents constitutes gross misconduct where it interferes with working practice.

i) Alcohol drunk during working hours e.g. at leaving parties and at Christmas must be kept to an absolute minimum and it is the responsibility of each member of staff to be aware of his/her own ability to hold alcohol.

ii) Under no circumstances should an occupational therapist drive a patient on a home visit after consuming any alcohol.

iii) Staff arranging leaving parties or other celebrations should not encourage others to break this code by over provision of alcohol.

Principle
9. Personal profit/gain
Occupational therapists must not solicit for personal financial gain. They must not accept tokens such as favours, gifts or hospitality which might be construed as seeking to obtain preferential treatment.

Notes
Occupational therapists should adhere to the guidelines or procedures published by employing authorities which outline ways of dealing with gifts and donations. Occupational therapists in private practice should refer to the current British Association of Occupational Therapists' Guidelines on Private Practice.

i) Consumers do, from time to time, offer gifts to occupational therapists. Provided these are fairly small in nature and are not in the form of money, and if the occupational therapist feels the patient would be hurt by a refusal, it is permissible to accept. If the present is substantial, the therapist should explain to the consumer that this is outside the rules. When in doubt the supervisor should be consulted.

ii) Where a consumer offers to sell an object to an occupational therapist this should always be the subject of discussion between the occupational therapist and supervisor. Where the object has no obvious, reasonable price, an assessment of its value should be made by an appropriate third party and put in writing. The transaction, if agreed, should then be undertaken in clearly conducted terms and a written receipt obtained. This procedure should also be followed if selling an object to a consumer.

Principle
10. Advertising
BAOT members may make direct contact with potential referring employing agencies to promote their private practice. Display signs are a requirement and shall be dignified and restrained in character, and limited to such as are in position, size and wording no more than are reasonably required to indicate to persons seeking them the exact location of and entrance to the premises where the treatment is undertaken. It is necessary to comply with local bye-laws.

C. PROFESSIONAL RELATIONSHIPS AND RESPONSIBILITIES

Principle
11. Professional Demeanour
Occupational therapists must conduct themselves in a manner befitting professionals.

Notes
The profession is judged by the conduct and presentation of its members as they carry out their duties.

i) Any occupational therapist, in whichever field of speciality, shall present him/herself as a responsible, mature individual. The demeanour and personal presentation should inspire confidence and trust in the consumer.

Personal appearance will therefore be clean and the clothes appropriate to the clinical setting. All clothes must be clean and in good repair.

The general guideline of whether, in a time of crisis or difficulty, someone with your appearance and manner would inspire confidence in the client if your roles were reversed, should always be applied.

ii) Contacts with other professionals, agencies and the public will always be made in a courteous and positive manner.

iii) Uniforms should not normally be worn when off the hospital site, other than when this is on official business e.g. on a home visit. If uniform is worn off site on non-official business it should be covered by an outside garment.

Principle
12 Loyalty
Occupational therapists shall be loyal to fellow members of the profession and shall respect and uphold their dignity.

Notes
a) Any reference to the quality of service rendered by, or the integrity of a professional colleague will be expressed with due care to protect the reputation of that person.
b) Loyalty within any profession cannot eventually override one's responsibility as a member of society to uphold its moral and legal obligations. If an occupational therapist is in doubt over the fitness to practise of a colleague, he or she can appeal, in confidence, to the College of Occupational Therapists' Personal Advisory Panel.

i) If a therapist feels uncomfortable about the behaviour or professional performance of a colleague, of whatever discipline, this should be notified confidentially to the supervising occupational therapist, the head occupational therapist or district area occupational therapist or local authority equivalents, as appropriate.

ii) Under no circumstances must any occupational therapist, who witnesses malpractice, whether by an occupational therapist or other professional, remain silent about it. It must be reported immediately to a senior member of staff [see para. (i)], who will take appropriate action.

iii) The appropriate action for the senior member of staff is to investigate the allegation and seek an urgent discussion with the appropriate head of department.

Principle
13 Working relationships
Occupational therapists shall consult and co-operate with those with whom they come into contact during the course of their professional duties. Occupational therapists shall respect the needs, traditions, practices, special competencies, and responsibilities of their own and other professions, institutions and agencies that constitute their working environment.

Notes
Occupational therapists must protect the privacy of all those with whom they collaborate professionally. If an occupational therapist has first hand knowledge that a colleague's performance falls below reasonable standards, the therapist shall attempt to rectify the situation. Failing an informal solution, the occupational therapist shall use procedures established within the facility or agency to call the behaviour to the attention of management and use those procedures to handle such situations. Under no circumstances should the occupational therapist remain silent when the status of a consumer, student or organisation is in jeopardy.

D. PROFESSIONAL STANDARDS

Principle
14 Clinical competence
Occupational therapists must acknowledge the limits of their competence and experience. They shall only provide services and use techniques for which they are qualified by training and/or experience.

Notes
a) Occupational therapists shall recognise the value of regular appraisal and evaluation of the service they provide.
b) Occupational therapists who delegate treatment or other procedures must be satisfied that the person to whom these are delegated is competent to carry them out. Occupational therapists in these circumstances retain ultimate responsibility for the management of the consumer.
c) Occupational therapists should refrain from undertaking any activity in which problems or conflicts of a personal nature are likely to affect their competence or cause harm to patients, clients or colleagues.
d) Occupational therapists should recognise that a number of professions share common skills and thus their boundaries of practice may overlap.

i) Any occupational therapist who is asked to act up or cover for an absent colleague must identify any areas of work in which he/she does not feel competent.

ii) Occupational therapists working in areas that are unfamiliar or in which experience has not been recent should expect and can demand adequate supervision and support. If this is not forthcoming the therapist should notify the head occupational therapist or district/area occupational therapist or local authority equivalent, in writing.

iii) Occupational therapists should strive to identify their key roles in multidisciplinary team work. The teaching and advisory role should be recognised and used.

Principle
15 Referral of consumers

Occupational therapists shall undertake treatment either when the consumer has been referred by a medical practitioner or where occupational therapists have access to the consumer's doctor.

Notes
Health Circular (HC(77)333). 'Relationships between the Medical and Remedial Profession' is relevant.
  'Blanket referral' systems are appropriate provided medical clinicians are fully aware that this system exists.

Principle
16 Keeping records of consumers
Occupational therapists shall keep concise, factual records and reports for the information of professional colleagues and for legal purposes.

Notes
a) The Data Protection Act 1984 requires computerised records to contain facts only.
b) Provision must be made for the secure and confidential storage and disposal of records. Refer to local procedures.
c) Refer to NHS code of practice on access to personal health information and Local Authority procedures on consumer access.
d) All records are required to be kept for a statutory length of time. Refer to Health Circular (HC(80)7).

i) Every consumer shall have an up to date record containing :-
*personal history as appropriate
*medical history
assessment of ability/disability
objectives of treatment
timescale for achieving objectives/goals (if possible)
outline of treatment methodology
copies of reports and letters.
These records must be regularly updated and achievements and treatment reviewed.

ii) Entries into a consumer's notes shall be made not later than the following working day after the consumer contact and preferably the same day. Significant phone calls should also be entered.
  The exception to this frequency of recording may be for longer term consumers, where regular reviews/progress should be documented at least monthly, or in exceptional cases to a time-scale agreed with the therapist line manager.

iii) Wherever possible, occupational therapy written records and notes should be with the consumer's main note file. Where not possible, easily identifiable reference to occupational therapy involvement must be contained in the main notes.

iv) Notes shall not contain subjective opinion that cannot be substantiated. Care must be taken over terminology used to ensure that it corresponds with facts presented.

*Where adequate/appropriate information is contained in the consumer's main notes, this should be in precis form only or reference made to the facts contained therein.

Principle
17 Professional development
Occupational therapists shall be responsible for actively maintaining and developing personal professional competence.

Occupational therapists shall promote:-
• an understanding of and research into occupational therapy.
• the education of students and colleagues.

Notes
a) All members of the occupational therapy profession have an individual responsibility to maintain their level of professional competence and each must strive to improve and update knowledge and skills.

b) Occupational therapists must always share their professional expertise with and disseminate it to, fellow professionals, colleagues and students.

c) Members of the profession shall promote understanding of occupational therapy to the general public.

d) Occupational therapists have a responsibility to contribute to the continuing development of the profession by critical evaluation and research. Any research undertaking has additional ethical implications which occupational therapists must respect.

e) Occupational therapists shall acquire knowledge about local and national issues as they affect the occupational therapy profession.

f) The Professions Supplementary to Medicine Act 1960 bestows the status of a profession on occupational therapy which automatically carries the statutory requirement to regulate professional practice for the protection of patients or clients.

i) The maintenance and development of professional standards is a requirement of continued practice. Occupational therapists must programme into their work schedule opportunities for reading and continued learning. The time allocated for this should be agreed with the head occupational therapist.

ii) Each occupational therapist should be responsible for maintaining a 'log book' of additional training education/learning received and undertaken. A record should also be kept of training courses applied for which were not successful due to lack of funding or unavailability of places.

iii) Occupational therapists should, with their supervisor, review the content of any training course undertaken and subsequently review its value to the competence of the occupational therapist concerned.

iv) As part of the appraisal/development process, occupational therapists should consider their personal and professional development and translate these into realistic yearly objectives, with a proposed implementation plan.

v) Research proposals and undertakings must adhere to international, national and local regulations.

APPENDIX H

The Scope of Professional Practice for Nurses, Midwifery and Health Visitors

INTRODUCTION
1. The practice of nursing, midwifery and health visiting requires the application of knowledge and the simultaneous exercise of judgement and skill. Practice takes place in a context of continuing change and development. Such change and development may result from advances in research leading to improvements in treatment and care, from alterations to the provision of health and social care services, as a result of changes in local policies and as a result of new approaches to professional practice. Practice must, therefore, be sensitive, relevant and responsive to the needs of individual patients and clients and have the capacity to adjust, where and when appropriate, to changing circumstances.

2. Education and experience form the foundation on which nurses, midwives and health visitors exercise judgement and skill, these, naturally, being developed and refined over time. The range of responsibilities which fall to individual nurses, midwives and health visitors should be related to their personal experience, education and skill. This range or responsibilities is described here as the 'scope of professional practice' and this paper sets out the Council's principles on which any adjustment to the scope of professional practice should be based. The contents of this paper are set out on page 2.

Education for Professional Practice
3. Just as practice must remain dynamic, sensitive, relevant and responsive to the changing needs of patients and clients, so too must education for practice. Pre-registration education prepares nurses, midwives and health visitors for safe practice at the point of registration. The pre-registration curriculum will continue to change over time to absorb relevant changes in care as advances are made. Pre-registration education is, therefore, a foundation for professional practice and a means of equipping nurses, midwives and health visitors with the necessary knowledge and skills to assume responsibility as registered practitioners. This foundation education alone, however, cannot effectively meet the changing and complex demands of the range of modern health care. Post-registration education equips practitioners with additional and more specialist skills necessary to meet the special needs of patients and clients. There is a broad range of post-registration provision and the Council regards adequate and effective provision of quality education as a prerequisite of quality care.

Registration and the Code of Professional Conduct for the Nurse, Midwife and Health Visitor
4. The act of registration by the Council confers on individual nurses, midwives and health visitors the legal right to practise and to use the title 'registered'. From the point of registration, each practitioner is subject to the Council's Code of Professional Conduct and accountable for his or her practice and conduct. The Code provides a statement of the values of the professions and establishes the framework within which

practitioners practise and conduct themselves. The act of registration and the expectations stated in the Code are central to the Council's key role in regulating the standards of the professions in the interest of patients and clients and of society as a whole.

5. Once registered, each nurse, midwife and health visitor remains subject to the Code and ultimately accountable to the Council for his or her actions and omissions. This position applies regardless of the employment circumstances and regardless of whether or not individuals are actively engaged in practice. This position will only change if the decision is made by the Council (through clearly established legal processes related to professional misconduct or unfitness to practise due to illness) to remove a name from the Council's register. This reflects the key, central role which the registration process plays in maintaining standards in the public interest. On the specific question of employment of nurses in the personal social services in general and the residential care sector in particular, the Council recognises that there are ambiguities. These are addressed in paragraphs 20 and 21 of this paper.

The Code of Professional Conduct and the Scope of Professional Practice
6. The Code includes a number of explicit clauses which relate to changes to the scope of practice in nursing, midwifery and health visiting. These clauses are :

'As a registered nurse, midwife or health visitor you are personally accountable for your practice and, in the exercise of your professional accountability, must:

6.1   act always in such a manner as to promote and safeguard the interests and well-being of patients and clients;
    6.2   ensure that no action or omission on your part, or within your sphere of responsibility, is detrimental to the interests, condition or safety of patients and clients;

6.3   maintain and improve your professional knowledge and competence;

6.4   acknowledge any limitations in your knowledge and competence, and decline any duties or responsibilities unless able to perform them in a safe and skilled manner.

7. The Code, therefore, provides a firm bedrock upon which decisions about adjustments to the scope of professional practice can be made. There are, however, important distinctions relating to the scope of practice in nursing, in midwifery and in health visiting. These are described in the paragraphs that follow the Council's principles for adjusting the scope of practice. These principles apply to the practice of nursing, midwifery and health visiting addressed later in this paper and to any application of complementary or alternative and other therapies by nurses, midwives or health visitors.

Principles for adjusting the Scope of Practice
8. Although the practices of nursing, midwifery and health visiting differ widely, the same principles apply to the scope of practice in each of these professions. The following principles are based upon the Council's Code of Professional Conduct and, in particular, on the emphasis which the Code places upon knowledge, skill,

responsibility and accountability. The principles which should govern adjustments to the scope of professional practice are those which follow:

9. The registered nurse, midwife or health visitor:

9.1   must be satisfied that each aspect of practice is directed to meeting the needs and serving the interests of the patient or client;

9.2   must endeavour always to achieve, maintain and develop knowledge, skill and competence to respond to those needs and interests;

9.3   must honestly acknowledge any limits of personal knowledge and skill and take steps to remedy any relevant deficits in order effectively and appropriately to meet the needs of patients and clients;

9.4   must ensure that any enlargement or adjustment of the scope of personal professional practice must be achieved without compromising or fragmenting existing aspects of professional practice and care and that the requirements of the Council's Code of Professional Conduct are satisfied throughout the whole area of practice;

95.   must recognise and honour the direct or indirect personal accountability borne for all aspects of professional practice and

9.6   must, in serving the interests of patients and clients and the wider interests of society, avoid any inappropriate delegation to others which compromises those interests.

10.   These principles for practice should enhance trust and confidence within a health care team and promote further the important collaborative work between medical and nursing, midwifery and health visiting practitioners upon which good practice and care depends.

11.   The Council recognises that care by registered nurses, midwives and health visitors is provided in health care, social care and domestic settings. Patients and clients require skilled care from registered practitioners and support staff require direction and supervision from these same practitioners. These matters are directly concerned with standards of care. This paper, therefore, also addresses the matter of the 'identified' practitioner, practice in the personal social services and residential care sector and support for professional practice.

The Scope and 'Extended Practice' of Nursing
12.   The practice of nursing has traditionally been based on the premise that pre-registration education equips the nurse to perform at a certain level and to encompass a particular range of activities. It is also based on the premise that any widening of that range and enhancement of the nurse's practice requires 'official' extension of that role by certification.

13.   The Council considers that the terms 'extended' or 'extending' roles which have been associated with this system are no longer suitable since they limit, rather than extend, the parameters or practice. As a result, many practitioners have been prevented from fulfilling their potential for the benefit of patients. The Council also believes that a concentration on 'activities' can detract from the importance of holistic nursing care. The Council has therefore determined the principles set out in paragraphs 8-10 inclusive to provide the basis for ensuring that practice remains dynamic and is able readily and appropriately to adjust to meet changing care needs.

14.   The reality is that the practice of nursing and education for that practice will continue to be shaped by developments in care and treatment, and by other events which influence it. This equally applies to midwifery and health visiting. In order to bring into proper focus the professional responsibility and consequent accountability of individual practitioners, it is the Council's principles for practice rather than certificates for tasks which should form the basis for adjustments to the scope of practice.

The Scope of Midwifery Practice

15   The position in relation to midwifery practice is set out in the Council's Midwife's Code of Practice. This indicates that it is the individual midwife's responsibility to maintain and develop the competence which she has acquired during her training, recognising the sphere of practice in which she is deemed to be equipped to practise with safety and competence. It also indicates that, while some developments in midwifery become an essential and integral part of the role of every midwife (and are subsequently incorporated into pre-registration education), other developments may require particular midwives to acquire new skills because of the particular settings in which they are practising. The importance of local policies which are in accord with the Council's policies and standards and the guidelines issued by the National Boards for Nursing, Midwifery and Health Visiting is self-evident. The importance of the midwife practising outside the area of her employing authority or outside the National Health Service discussing the full scope of her practice with her supervisor of midwives is emphasised in the Midwife's Code of Practice.

16.   It can be seen from this position that it is accepted by the Council that some developments in midwifery care can become an integral part of the role of all midwives and other developments may become part of the role of some midwives. The Council believes that the Midwife's Code of Practice, cited above, and the Code of Professional Conduct, together provide key principles to underpin the scope of midwifery practice. These are now supplemented by those stated in paragraphs 8 to 10 inclusive of this paper.

The Scope of Health Visiting Practice

17.   The position of health visiting differs from that of nursing and midwifery, as there are frequent occasions when the full contribution of health visitors may not find expression where it is most needed. There is, for example, often a concentration on the role of the health visitor in relation to those in the under-five age group at the expense of other groups in the community who need, and would benefit from the special preparation and skill of health visitors. These circumstances have the effect

of constraining practice and limiting the degree to which individuals and communities are able to benefit from the knowledge and skill of health visitors. There is merit in allowing health visitors, where they judge it to be appropriate, to use the full range of their skills in response to needs identified in the pursuit of their health visiting practice. To single out any aspect of practice would be unwise but, where health and nursing need is identified, the health visitor is well placed to determine what intervention may be necessary and able to draw on both her nursing and health visiting education.

18.   The community setting of health visiting practice, the relationship between numerous agencies and services and the health visitor's professional relationship with clients and their families are factors which must be taken into consideration. The health visitor, in all aspects of her practice, is subject to the Council's Code of Professional Conduct and should also satisfy the requirements of paragraphs 8 to 10 inclusive of this paper.

Practice and the 'Identified' Nurse, Midwife and Health Visitor
19.   The Council recognises that, in a growing number of settings, patients and clients will be in the care of an 'identified' practitioner. The practitioner may be identified as the 'named' practitioner or as the primary, associate or sole practitioner providing nursing, midwifery or health visiting care. In such roles, individuals assume key responsibility for coordinating and supervising the delivery of care, drawing on the general and special resources of colleagues where appropriate. Professional Practice naturally involves recognising and accepting accountability for these matters. The Council expects that practitioners will recognise the need to provide all necessary support for colleagues and ensure that practice is underpinned by the required knowledge and skill. The Council equally expects that practitioners identified in one of these ways will be fully prepared for, and supported, in this key role.

Practice in the Personal Social Services and Residential Care Sector
20.   The Council recognises that the community nursing services have a duty to provide a nursing service to those in need of nursing care in the personal social services and residential care sector. Registered nurses who are employed in this sector, whether in homes or in the provision of other services, remain accountable to the Council and subject to the Council's Code of Professional Conduct, even if their posts do not require nursing qualifications. In this regard, as explained in paragraph 5 of this paper, the position of such nurses is the same as that of nurses engaged in direct professional nursing practice.

21.   The Council requires that registered nurses employed in such circumstances will use their judgement and discretion to identify the nursing needs of residents and others for whom they may have responsibility, and will comply with any requirements of the Council. The Council expects that employers will recognise the advantages to the personal social services and residential care sector which result from the employment of registered nurses.

Support for Professional Practice

22.   Nurses, midwives and health visitors require support in their work. In institutional and community settings, a range of support staff form part of the team. The development of the health care assistant role is linked with a form of vocational training. The Council does not have a direct role in this training, but recognises that this development has an impact upon aspects of care and on the practice and standard of nursing, midwifery and health visiting, for which the Council is responsible.

23.   The Council's position in relation to support roles is as follows :

23.1 health care assistants to registered nurses, midwives and health visitors must work under the direction and supervision of those registered practitioners;

23.2 registered nurses, midwives and health visitors must remain accountable for assessment, planning and standards of care and for determining the activity of their support staff;

23.3 health care assistants must not be allowed to work beyond their level of competence;

23.4 continuity of care and appropriate skill/staff mix is important, so health care assistants should be integral members of the caring team;

23.5 standards of care must be safeguarded and the need for patients and clients, across the spectrum of health care, to receive skilled professional nursing, midwifery and health visiting assessment and care must be recognised as of primary importance;

23.6 health care assistants with the desire and ability to progress to professional education should be encouraged to obtain vocational qualifications, some of which may be approved by the Council as acceptable entry criteria into programmes of professional education and

23.7 registered nurses, midwives and health visitors should be involved in these developments so that the support role can be designed to ensure that professional skills are used most appropriately for the benefit of patients and clients.

Conclusion

24.   The principles set out in paragraphs 8 to 10 inclusive of this paper should form the basis for any decisions relating to adjustments to the scope of practice. These principles should replace the system of certification for specific tasks. They provide a realistic, effective and rational approach to adjustments to professional practice.

25.   This change has consequences for managers of clinical practice and professional leaders of nursing, midwifery and health visiting, who must ensure that local policies and procedures are based upon the principles set out in this paper and in the Council's Code of Professional Conduct. Any local arrangements must ensure that registered nurses, midwives and health visitors are assisted to undertake, and are enabled to fulfil, any suitable adjustments to their scope of practice.

26.   This statement sets out the Council's position relating to the scope of professional practice of the professions it regulates, to the 'identified' practitioner, to practice in the residential care sector and to support staff. The Council hopes that this statement, and the principles which it sets out will provide a clear framework for the logical and desirable development of practice and for the management of practice and care teams. The framework provides for greater flexibility in practice and for enhancing the contribution to care of nurses, midwives and health visitors. Above all, the framework and the principles reflect the personal responsibility and accountability of individual practitioners, entrusted by the Council to protect and improve standards of care.

A UKCC Position Paper, June 1992.

Reproduced by kind permission of the UKCC.

APPENDIX I

Confidentiality

Summary of the principles on which to base professional judgement in matters of confidentiality.

1. That a patient/client has a right to expect that information given in confidence will be used only for the purpose for which it was given and will not be released to others without their consent.

2. That practitioners recognise the fundamental right of their patients/clients to have information about them held in secure and private storage.

3. That, where it is deemed appropriate to share information obtained in the course of professional practice with other health or social work practitioners, the practitioner who obtained the information must ensure, as far as is reasonable, before its release that it is being imparted in strict professional confidence and for a specific purpose.

4. That the responsibility to either disclose or withhold confidential information in the public interest lies with the individual practitioner, that he/she cannot delegate the decision, and that he/she cannot be required by a superior to disclose or withhold information against his/her will.

5. That a practitioner who chooses to breach the basic principle of confidentiality in the belief that it is necessary in the public interest must have considered the matter sufficiently to justify that decision.

6. That deliberate breaches of confidentiality, other than with the consent of the patient/client should be exceptional.

A UKCC Advisory Paper, April, 1987.

Reproduced by kind permission of the UKCC.

APPENDIX J

Exercising Accountability

(UKCC Advisory Document, March 1989).

SUMMARY OF THE PRINCIPLES AGAINST WHICH TO EXERCISE ACCOUNTABILITY
1. The interests of the patient or client are paramount.

2. Professional accountability must be exercised in such a manner as to ensure that the primacy of the interests of patients or clients is respected and must not be overridden by those of the professions or their practitioners.

3. The exercise of accountability requires the practitioner to seek to achieve and maintain high standards.

4. Advocacy on behalf of patients or clients is an essential feature of the exercise of accountability by a professional practitioner.

5. The role of other persons in the delivery of health care to patients or clients must be recognised and respected, provided that the first principle above is honoured.

6. Public trust and confidence in the profession is dependent on the practitioners being seen to exercise their accountability responsibly.

7. Each registered nurse, midwife or health visitor must be able to justify any action or decision not to act taken in the course of her professional practice.

A UKCC Advisory Document, March 1989.
Reproduced by kind permission of the UKCC.

APPENDIX K

The Patient's Charter

SEVEN EXISTING RIGHTS:
Every citizen already has the following National Health Service rights:

1. To receive health care on the basis of clinical need, regardless of ability to pay.

2. To be registered with a GP.

3. To receive emergency medical care at any time, through your GP or the emergency ambulance service and hospital accident and emergency department.

4. To be referred to a consultant, acceptable to you, when your GP thinks it necessary and to be referred for a second opinion if you and your GP agree this is desirable.

5. To be given a clear explanation of any treatment proposed, including any risks and any alternatives, before you decide whether you will agree to the treatment.

6. To have access to your health records, and to know that those working for the NHS will, by law, keep their contents confidential.

7. To choose whether or not you wish to take part in medical research or medical student training.

THREE NEW RIGHTS
From 1 April 1992, you will have three important new rights:

1. To be given detailed information on local health services, including quality standards and maximum waiting times. You will be able to get this information from your health authority, GP or Community Health Council.

2. To be guaranteed admission for virtually all treatments by a specific date no later than two years from the day when your consultant places you in a waiting list. Most patients will be admitted before this date. Currently, 90% are admitted within a year.

3. To have any complaint about NHS services - whoever provides them - investigated, and to receive a full and prompt written reply from the chief executive of your health authority or general manager of your hospital. If you are still unhappy, you will be able to take the case up with the Health Service Commissioner.

NATIONAL CHARTER STANDARDS
There are nine standards of service which the NHS will be aiming to provide for you:

1. Respect for privacy, dignity and religious and cultural belief.

2. Arrangements to ensure everyone, including people with special needs, can use the services.

3. Information to relatives and friends about the progress of your treatment, subject of course, to your wishes.

4. An emergency ambulance should arrive within 14 minutes in an urban area, or 19 minutes in a rural area.

5. When attending an accident and emergency department, you will be seen immediately and your need for treatment assessed.

6. When you go to an outpatient clinic, you will be given a specific appointment time and will be seen within 30 minutes of it.

7. Your operation should not be cancelled on the day you are due to arrive in hospital. If, exceptionally, your operation has to be postponed twice you will be admitted to hospital within one month of the second cancelled operation.

8. A named qualified nurse, midwife or health visitor responsible for your nursing or midwifery care.

9. A decision should be made about any continuing health or social care needs you may have, before you are discharged from hospital.

LOCAL CHARTER STANDARDS

In addition to National Charter Standards, there are many other aspects of the service which are important to you. From 1 April 1992, authorities will increasingly set and publicise clear Local Charter Standards, including:

1. First outpatient appointments.

2. Waiting times in accident and emergency departments, after initial assessment.

3. Waiting times for taking you home after treatment, where your doctor says you have a medical need for NHS transport.

4. Enabling you and your visitors to find your way around hospitals, through enquiry points and better signposting.

5. Ensuring that the staff you meet face to face wear name badges.

Reproduced by kind permission of The Department of Health.

APPENDIX L

British Medical Association (BMA) Guidelines

The BMA has published a series of invaluable guidelines/proposals which address both the ethical and legal aspects of decision making in a number of situations which can arise in practice. Some guidelines have been developed as a collaborative exercise with other professional bodies such as the Royal College of Nursing. These guidelines, which are strongly recommended to readers of this text, are published in leaflet form and are available on application to the Publications Section of the BMA, BMA House, Tavistock Square, London WC1H 9JR. A summary of some of the key content areas incorporated in these guidelines which are relevant to be ethical and legal issues explored in this text is provided below. This summary does not cover the range of BMA guidelines available.

1. Decisions Related to Cardiopulmonary Resuscitation (CPR).
   Collaborative Paper (BMA, RCN, Resuscitation Council).
   This paper considers the background to 'do not resuscitate' (DNR) orders and situations when it appropriate to consider DNR decisions. The overall responsibility for such decisions is identified as lying with the medical consultant. This responsibility is discussed in relation to individuals involved in decision making and other wide-ranging factors which must be considered. These include express wishes of the patient; the family (addressing confidentiality); decision making involving the medical/nursing team. The contribution of factors such as the patient's medical condition, likelihood of success in CPR, and quality/duration of life are identified.
   The responsibility for decision making is considered apropos, understanding of policies by staff, discussion of decisions with other health professionals and the crucial need to review decisions in the light of changes in the patient's condition. Recommendations are made concerning documentation of DNR decisions in medical and nursing records.

2. Proposals for Establishment of a Decision Making Procedure on Behalf of the Mentally Incapable

These proposals explore the issues and mechanisms for obtaining valid consent to treatment/diagnostic procedures, when patients are incapable of a full understanding by virtue of mental illness of handicap. A key proposal is that each health district establishes a committee (membership recommended) to provide a mechanism through which decision making in relation to valid consent can be obtained.
   Levels of decision making are stratified at three levels, covering simple treatments/diagnostic procedures which involve minimal risk, to those which can result in serious risk to life. The role of the committee in delegating decisions (within defined limits) in certain situations is noted. The proposals also suggest that the Mental Health Act Commissioners could offer such a Committee guidance and support in fulfilling its function and also act in a supervisory capacity.

3. Guidelines for Doctors on the Access to Health Records Act 1990.

These comprehensive guidelines cover the historical background to information access in the light of patients' expectations, medical roles, and the content of other statutory acts such as the Data Protection Act 1984. Consideration is given to safeguards which must be employed on behalf of patients and health professions in relation to access. Rights of access, the scope of information which can be disclosed/not disclosed, eligibility to apply, procedures to be employed, amendments, fees and appeals to the Courts are all succinctly reviewed. Clear and concise advice is given concerning record keeping by health professionals.

4. Medical Treatment and Incapable Adults

These guidelines consider the issue of informed consent in adults who are incapable of giving consent to medical treatment. From a legal perspective, situations where treatment can be given without consent due to impaired capacity are identified (ie. impaired maturity, consciousness, mental disorder leading to behaviour constituting a serious danger, detention under the Mental Health Act). Emphasis is placed on the fundamental precept that what is in the patient's best interest (criteria identified) directs treatment in all cases. Examples of exceptional circumstances in which proposed treatments should not be carried out without High Court approval are described.

In relation to the assessment of patients' capacity to make decisions about their treatment, basic principles which, in addition to clinical, professional and legal factors, could guide such an assessment are identified. Emphasis is also placed in these guidelines on the need not to lose sight of the principle/duty of confidentiality in treatment decisions/discussions with relatives/caregivers, courts, government agencies and others.

The rights of patients identified as being incapable of giving informed consent to treatment are summarised, ie. those related to freedom from discrimination, respect for privacy, confidentiality, dignity and to be free from medical treatments which exert a negative impact on quality of life. The need to consider the patients' views about treatment is emphasised despite legal incapacity to consent. The guidelines also discuss the issue of treatment safeguards and propose procedures to be observed for serious treatments. Guidelines are also included which address the issue of participation by incapacitated individuals in therapeutic research studies.

5. Decisions for Patients in a Persistent Vegetative State (PVS)

This paper summarises the background to ethical and legal issues related to implementing and withdrawing treatment for individual suffering from PVS. The importance of an initial assessment and treatment are emphasised, in conjunction with the need to provide aggressive medical therapy at this stage. A recommendation is made that a diagnosis of PVS is not confirmed until the individual has been insentient for 12 months, and that a decision to withdraw treatment should only be considered after this period. The need for independent medical opinion to be employed in relation to the latter is noted. The need for a range of factors to be considered in relation to decisions concerning treatment options is emphasised. These include the views of the patient (advance directives); those close to the patient medical/health professional's views; legal issues; diagnosis/prognosis and benefits versus burdens of treatment. These guidelines note the acceptability in some circumstances of withdrawing treatment in the patient's best interest and requirements for legal consultation in such cases.

Index